PSYCHOLOGY, MENTAL HEALTH
AND YOGA

Psychology, Mental Health and Yoga

Essays on

SRI AUROBINDO'S PSYCHOLOGICAL THOUGHT
IMPLICATIONS OF YOGA FOR MENTAL HEALTH

THIRD EDITION

A. S. DALAL

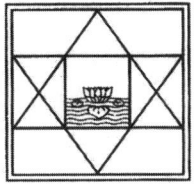

INSTITUTE OF INTEGRAL YOGA PSYCHOLOGY
INDIA

This book was first published by Sri Aurobindo Ashram Press,
    Pondicherry, 1991
Reprinted: 1992, 1996, 2000
A second edition (revised and enlarged) was printed in 2001

First Auroshakti Foundation edition 2012

Rs. 120.00
ISBN 978-81-924477-0-4

        Lotus Press
        PO Box 325
Twin Lakes, WI 53181 USA
   www.lotuspress.com
 lotuspress@lotuspress.com

CONTENTS

Preface to the First Edition ... vii
Notes on the Second and the Third Edition ... ix

PART ONE
PSYCHOLOGY AND YOGA

1. Sri Aurobindo and Modern Psychology ... 3
2. Sri Aurobindo and the Concept of the Unconscious in Psychology ... 24
3. Self-Awareness in Psychology and Sri Aurobindo's Yoga ... 46
4. The Nature of Identification ... 58

PART TWO
MENTAL HEALTH AND YOGA

5. Mental Health and Sri Aurobindo's Integral Yoga ... 71
6. Jung on the Suitability of Yoga for the West: A Critique in the Light of Sri Aurobindo's Thought ... 85
7. Psychological Disturbances: A Model Based on Sri Aurobindo's Thought ... 96
8. Attitudes, Mental Health and Yoga ... 122
9. Mastery, Mental Health and Yoga ... 132
10. The Healing Power of Peace ... 144

Index ... 157

PREFACE TO THE FIRST EDITION

The essays brought together in this book appeared at first in the annual numbers of *Sri Aurobindo Circle* between 1983 and 1990. Since the essays were written as independent articles published at long intervals rather than as a connected and closely-knit series, several ideas and references to literature, including quotations, were repeated. In the present collection of the essays undue repetitions have been removed wherever this could be done wihout major revisions.

Since the birth of modern psychology a little over a hundred years ago, views regarding the nature of the human being have followed a certain progressive trend which may be conceived as a dimensional development. Psychology began with a lateral view of the human being as an essentially animal organism capable of certain superior psychological functions which have generally been labelled as "mind". To this surface view was added a new dimension by the "depth" psychologies which discovered "the unconscious", ascribing to it a greater role than the conscious mind in determining behaviour. During the past few decades, yet another dimension — that of "height" — has been discovered through experiences of "higher" states of consciousness which have been termed "transpersonal". With this dimensional progression of views about the human constitution, psychology has been drawing increasingly closer to the pluridimensional concept of the human being found in yoga. Since notions of mental health stem from theories regarding personality structure, the emerging convergence of psychology and yoga is reflected also in the field of mental health. The purpose of this book is to present some salient features of Sri Aurobindo's psychological thought and its implications for mental health in order to bring out some points of convergence, as also of divergence, between psychology and mental health on the one hand, and yoga on the other.

Three main categories of readers have been kept in view in writing these essays: students and practitioners of Sri Aurobindo's yoga who have an interest in modern psychology and in what today goes by the name of mental health; secondly, students and teachers of psychology who wish to have an introduction to Sri Aurobindo's psychological thought and its bearing on mental health; finally, persons interested in the interface between modern psychology and mental health on the one hand and yoga on the other — yoga construed broadly as a consciousness discipline, that is, as a psycho-transformative system for the attainment of a more evolved state of consciousness.

The essays utilise copious quotations from the works of Sri Aurobindo and the Mother in giving an exposition of the psychological thought of their yoga. These actual words of the Masters have an intuitive quality and are therefore capable of imparting something more than an intellectual understanding of yoga psychology. If read with a quiet concentration, they may enable the reader to sense something of their intuitive content which would be all but completely lost by paraphrasing the words. In this respect, the reader may find that the words of the Mother, though translated from French, are particularly helpful in inducing a certain receptive state which is conducive to a deeper understanding of what the words express, for, consisting mostly of her spoken utterances, they are less intellectually couched and let through their intuitive quality more readily.

NOTE ON THE SECOND EDITION

In this (enlarged and slightly revised) edition of the book, some additional extracts from the writings of Sri Aurobindo have been incorporated in the first two essays. The present edition also includes two new essays: "Mental Health and Sri Aurobindo's Integral Yoga" and "Jung on the Suitability of Yoga for the West: A Critique in the Light of Sri Aurobindo's Thought". The former essay was first published in *Sri Aurobindo Circle* (38th Number, 1982). The latter article is being published for the first time. Only a few minor revisions have been made in some of the essays. The chief revision will be found in the essay on "Sri Aurobindo and the Concept of the Unconscious in Psychology" in which the comparison between Jung's concept of the collective unconscious and Sri Aurobindo's concept of the subliminal has been further elaborated.

NOTE ON THE THIRD EDITION

The first essay, entitled "Sri Aurobindo and Modern Psychology", has been expanded and made more comprehensive. It now includes almost everything that Sri Aurobindo has said directly about modern psychology in his different works. The text of the essay has been recast so as to bring out more clearly Sri Aurobindo's views as they bear on each of the various schools of modern psychology. In particular, some of the chief similarities and differences between Sri Aurobindo and Carl Jung have been stated more explicitly in the present edition of the book.

PART ONE

PSYCHOLOGY AND YOGA

Yoga is nothing but practical psychology.

SRI AUROBINDO

Psychology without yoga is lifeless.
The study of psychology must necessarily lead to yoga, at least to practical yoga if not theoretical.

THE MOTHER

1 SRI AUROBINDO AND MODERN PSYCHOLOGY

Early Psychology

In the West, where modern psychology was born and cradled, psychological thought had for centuries been part of philosophical enquiry into the nature of the human being. As such, psychology was a handmaiden of philosophy. The emergence of psychology as an independent field of study in its own right and as an empirical science is generally traced to the founding of the first laboratory of experimental psychology by the German physiologist, Wilhelm Wundt, in Leipzig in 1879. During its earliest stage, psychology overshadowed by the natural sciences, developed strictly as a laboratory science, becoming what has been described as a "brass-instrument psychology". It studied relatively superficial aspects of behaviour, such as reaction time, conditioned reflexes, perceptual functions, attention span, localization of functions in the brain, and other similar areas of psychology which border on physiology. Alluding to this early psychology, Sri Aurobindo observed in 1916:

> Modern Science, obsessed with the greatness of its physical discoveries and the idea of the sole existence of Matter, has long attempted to base upon physical data even its study of Soul and Mind and of those workings of Nature in man and animal in which a knowledge of psychology is as important as any of the physical sciences. Its very psychology founded itself upon physiology and the scrutiny of the brain and nervous system.[1]

The earliest school of modern psychology called Structuralism (also sometimes referred to as Introspectionism), closely associated with the work of Edward B. Titchnener (1867-1927), tried to discover through experiment and introspective analysis the "elements of consciousness". Sri Aurobindo was most probably alluding to this earliest school of Structuralism when he wrote:

> ...it was a crude, scholastic and superficial systematization of man's ignorance of himself. The surface psychological functionings, will, mind, senses, reason, conscience, etc., were arranged in a dry and sterile classification; their real nature and relation to each other were not fathomed....[2]

Commenting on the superficial nature of early psychology and the need to look deeper in order to understand the true nature of consciousness, Sri Aurobindo wrote:

> ... psychological enquiry in Europe (and without enquiry there can be no sound knowledge) is only beginning and has not gone very far, and what has reigned in men's minds up to now is a superficial statement of the superficial appearances of our consciousness as they look to us at first view and nothing more. But knowledge only begins when we get away from the surface phenomena and look behind them for their true operations and causes. To the superficial view of the outer mind and senses the sun is a little fiery ball circling in mid air round the earth and the stars twinkling little things stuck in the sky for our benefit at night. Scientific enquiry comes and knocks this infantile first-view to pieces. The sun is a huge affair (millions of miles away from our air) around which the small earth circles, and the stars are huge members of huge systems indescribably distant which have nothing apparently to do with the tiny earth and her creatures. All Science is like that, a contradiction of the sense-view or superficial appearances of things and an assertion of truths which are unguessed by the common and the uninstructed reason. The same process has to be followed in psychology if we are really to know what our consciousness is, how it is built and made and what is the secret of its functionings or the way out of its disorder.[3]

Psychoanalysis — The First Force

The first systematic attempt to "get away from the surface phenomena and look behind them for their true operations and causes" was made by Psychoanalysis founded by Sigmund Freud (1856-1939). The mind, said Freud, is like an iceberg, of which nine-tenths — which he called the unconscious — lies below the surface of the conscious mind, therefore is inaccessible to introspection, and yet is the most powerful determinant and real cause of outward behaviour. Hailing the new "depth psychology" of the psychoanalytical school as an advancement upon the earlier psychology which dealt with only the surface mind, Sri Aurobindo stated:

> ... whatever the crudities of the new science, it has at least taken the first capital step without which there can be no true psychological knowledge; it has made the discovery which is the beginning of self-knowledge and which all must make who deeply study the facts of consciousness, that our waking and surface existence is only a small part of our being and does not yield to us the root and secret of our character, our mentality or our actions. The sources lie deeper. To discover them, to know the nature and the processes of the inconscient or subconscient self and, so far as is possible, to possess and utilise them as physical science possesses and utilises the secret of the forces of Nature, ought to be the aim of a scientific psychology.[4]

Some of Freud's views regarding the nature of what he labelled as the unconscious are strikingly corroborated in the following description of what in Sri Aurobindo's yoga is termed the subconscient:

> In our yoga we mean by the subconscient that quite submerged part of our being in which there is no wakingly conscious and coherent thought, will or feeling or organized reaction, but which yet receives obscurely the impressions of all things and

stores them up in itself and from it too all sorts of stimuli, of persistent habitual movements, crudely repeated or disguised in strange forms can surge up into dream or into the waking nature. For if these impressions rise up most in dream in an incoherent and disorganized manner, they can also and do rise up into our waking consciousness as a mechanical repetition of old thoughts, old mental, vital and physical habits or an obscure stimulus to sensations, actions, emotions which do not originate in or from our conscious thought or will and are even often opposed to its perceptions, choice or dictates. In the subconscient there is an obscure mind full of obstinate Sanskaras*[1], impressions, associations, fixed notions, habitual reactions formed by our past, an obscure vital full of the seeds of habitual desires, sensations and nervous reactions, a most obscure material which governs much that has to do with the condition of the body. It is largely responsible for our illnesses; chronic or repeated illnesses are indeed mainly due to the subconscient and its obstinate memory and habit of repetition of whatever has impressed itself upon the body-consciousness.[5]

The following are the chief Freudian views about the unconscious which reflect what Sri Aurobindo has stated about the subconscient*[2]:
  (a) The unconscious is far more extensive than the conscious.
  (b) What is repressed or driven out of conscious awareness becomes part of the unconscious.
  (c) The contents of the unconscious powerfully affect the workings of the conscious mind.
  (d) What lies in the unconscious emerges in dreams. (Dreams, said Freud, are the royal road to the unconscious.)

*[1] Associations, impressions, habitual reactions formed by one's past. (Author's note)

*[2] It should be noted that Sri Aurobindo distinguishes between the subconscient and what he calls the Inconscient. The latter, for which there is no equivalent in modern psychology, is the most involved state of consciousness, below even the subconscient.

(e) Certain experiences rooted in the unconscious tend to be re-enacted repeatedly in a compulsive way — what Freud termed "repetition compulsion".

The "crudities of the new science", spoken of earlier by Sri Aurobindo, arise from its extremely narrow conception of what it calls the unconscious. All that is outside the conscious awareness is attributed by Freud to the unconscious which is viewed chiefly as a storehouse of instincts and impulses, predominantly the sexual instinct, to which Freud assigned an exclusive role in the motivation of all normal as well as abnormal human behaviours — an infant's sucking reflex no less than literary and religious pursuits as well as the aberrations of hysteria and psychosis. What lies outside our conscious awareness, says Sri Aurobindo, is an unimaginably vast field of consciousness consisting of many parts and levels of being which are: *below* conscious awareness (the subconscient), *behind* it (the subliminal), and *above* it (the superconscient). Further, within each of these major divisions of the being there are many subdivisions.*[3] From this viewpoint, what Freud calls the unconscious is only a small part of the totality of our being. Consequently, in explaining all human behaviours in terms of this miniscule (though highly predominant) part — what Sri Aurobindo describes as the lower subconscient vital layer of the human being — psychoanalysis commits two related errors, namely, over-generalisation and reductionism.

Regarding the over-generalisation of psychoanalysis, Sri Aurobindo states:

> It [psychoanalysis of Freud] takes up a certain part, the darkest, the most perilous, the unhealthiest part of the nature, the lower vital subconscious layer, isolates some of its most morbid phenomena and attributes to it and them an action out of all proportion to its true role in the nature. Modern psychology is an infant science, at once rash, fumbling and crude. As in all infant sciences, the universal habit of the human mind — to

---

*[3] For a more detailed presentation of the subject, see "Sri Aurobindo and the Concept of the Unconscious in Psychology", the next essay in this book.

take a partial or local truth, generalise it unduly and try to explain a whole field of Nature in its narrow terms — runs riot here.[6]

The psychoanalytical error of reductionism is most prominent in explaining mystical and spiritual experiences in terms of the unconscious strivings of the id. In this regard, Sri Aurobindo remarks:

> I find it difficult to take these psycho-analysts at all seriously when they try to scrutinise spiritual experience by the flicker of their torch-lights, — yet perhaps one ought to, for half-knowledge is a powerful thing and can be a great obstacle to the coming in front of the true Truth. This new psychology looks to me very much like children learning some summary and not very adequate alphabet, exulting in putting their a-b-c-d of the subconscient and the mysterious underground super-ego together and imagining that their first book of obscure beginnings (c-a-t cat, t-r-e-e tree) is the very heart of the real knowledge. They look from down up and explain the higher lights by the lower obscurities; but the foundation of these things is above and not below, *upari budhna esam*.*[4] The super-conscient, not the subconscient, is the true foundation of things. The significance of the lotus is not to be found by analysing the secrets of the mud from which it grows here; its secret is to be found in the heavenly archetype of the lotus that blooms for ever in the Light above. The self-chosen field of these psychologists is besides poor, dark and limited; you must know the whole before you can know the part and the highest before you can truly understand the lowest. That is the promise of the greater psychology awaiting its hour before which these poor gropings will disappear and come to nothing.[7]

Psychoanalytical Treatment
Psychoanalysis stands for not only Freud's theory of personality and human behaviour but also for the method devised by him for

---

*[4] Their foundation is above (Rig Veda). (Author's note)

the study of the unconscious and the treatment of psychological disorders. As a method of treatment, psychoanalysis employs the interpretation of a person's free associations, dreams, fantasies, etc. in order to make conscious the unconscious underpinnings of the person's behaviour. Sri Aurobindo has pronounced on not only the psychoanalytical theory as stated above, but also on the psychoanalytical method of treatment.

While endorsing Freud's finding that impulses which are repressed from consciousness lie in what in psychoanalysis is called the unconscious and can cause disorders, Sri Aurobindo states that this truth has been exaggerated by psychoanalysis.

> ...some things are suppressed in the ordinary life and remain lying in the nature, suppressed but not eliminated; they may rise up any day or they may express themselves in various nervous forms or other disorders of the mind or vital or body without it being evident what is their real cause. This has been recently discovered by European psychologists and much emphasised, even exaggerated in a new science called psychoanalysis.[8]

Sri Aurobindo regarded psychoanalysis as ill-advised for a practitioner of his yoga. He wrote to a disciple:

> Your practice of psycho-analysis was a mistake. It has, for the time at least, made the work of purification more complicated, not easier. The psycho-analysis of Freud is the last thing that one should associate with yoga. It takes up a certain part, the darkest, the most perilous, the unhealthiest part of the nature, the lower vital subconscious layer, isolates some of its most morbid phenomena and attributes to it and them an action out of all proportion to its true role in the nature. ... Moreover, the exaggeration of the importance of suppressed sexual complexes is a dangerous falsehood and it can have a nasty influence and tend to make the mind and vital more and not less fundamentally impure than before.
>
> It is true that the subliminal*[5] in man is the largest part of

his nature and has in it the secret of the unseen dynamisms which explain his surface activities. But the lower vital subconscious which is all that this psycho-analysis of Freud seems to know, — and even of that it knows only a few ill-lit corners, — is no more than a restricted and very inferior portion of the subliminal whole. The subliminal self stands behind and supports the whole superficial man; it has in it a larger and more efficient mind behind the surface mind, a larger and more powerful vital behind the surface vital, a subtler and freer physical consciousness behind the surface bodily existence. And above them it opens to higher superconscient as well as below them to lower subconscient ranges. If one wishes to purify and transform the nature, it is the power of these higher ranges to which one must open and raise to them and change by them both the subliminal and the surface being. Even this should be done with care, not prematurely or rashly, following a higher guidance, keeping always the right attitude; for otherwise the force that is drawn down may be too strong for an obscure and weak frame of nature. But to begin by opening up the lower subconscious, risking to raise up all that is foul or obscure in it, is to go out of one's way to invite trouble. First, one should make the higher mind and vital strong and firm and full of light and peace from above; afterwards one can open up or even dive into the subconscious with more safety and some chance of a rapid and successful change.[9]

---

*[5] The term "subliminal" is here used in the broad sense of *all* that lies outside the conscious awareness. As explained previously, the vast field of consciousness of which we are normally unconscious consists of: the subconscient (that which lies *below* conscious awareness); the subliminal proper (that which lies *behind* the surface consciousness); and the superconscient (that which is *above* our normal consciousness). "Subliminal" here covers all the three divisions of what is unconscious to the normal consciousness.

Carl G. Jung

Freud's dogmatism which assigned an exclusive role to the sexual drive and its associated dynamics in the motivation of all human behaviour led to the first two major rival offshoots of psychoanalysis — Individual Psychology developed by Alfred Adler (1870-1937) and Analytical Psychology formulated by Carl Jung (1875-1961). Adler regarded the urge for power, rather than the sexual urge, as the chief motivating factor underlying human behaviour. As for Jung, he differed from Freud chiefly in two respects. In the first place, Jung maintained that the libido is not a purely sexual drive, but a general "psychic-energy" or "life-instinct" (somewhat similar to Bergson's *élan vital*) which expresses itself in diverse forms, including the sexual urge. Secondly, Jung believed that besides the individual unconscious spoken of by Freud, there is a collective unconscious which is common to the human race as a whole. The collective unconscious, according to Jung, plays a far greater role in determining an individual's behaviour than the personal unconscious.

Jung's broader concept of the libido as a general instinctual energy is somewhat akin to what Sri Aurobindo has termed the vital, which he speaks of as follows:

> The vital is the Life-nature made up of desires, sensations, feelings, passions, energies of action, will of desire, reactions of the desire-soul in man and of all that play of possessive and other related instincts, anger, fear, greed, lust, etc., that belong to this field of the nature.[10]

It should be evident that Sri Aurobindo's concept of the vital is more inclusive than even Jung's broad concept of the libido. It connotes life-force in all its gradations, from the relatively grosser life-energy (called Prana in Indian philosophy) which animates plants, animals as well as human beings, to the more evolved forms of the vital such as instincts, feelings and emotions. Though compared to Freud's or Adler's views, Jung's view of the libido is closer to that of Sri Aurobindo, the relative truth of what Freud and Adler maintained is corroborated by Sri Aurobindo according to whom the three strongest motivating forces for the ordinary individual are power, wealth and sex.[11] (See footnote *6.)

In Jung's concept of the collective unconscious, too, we find some degree of concurrence between Jung and Sri Aurobindo; the Jungian concept of the collective unconscious reflects several aspects of what Sri Aurobindo describes as the subliminal. Thus:

(a) In the subliminal, states Sri Aurobindo, are inner senses of sight, touch, hearing, etc.; the subliminal is therefore "the seer of inner things and supraphysical experiences".[12] Similarly, Jung, who reports having had frequent supraphysical experiences such as visions or what he called "extremely vivid hypnagogic images",[13] ascribed such experiences to the collective unconscious.

(b) Another striking resemblance between Sri Aurobindo's description of the subliminal and Jung's view of the collective unconscious lies in tracing the source of predictive, veridical and deeply symbolic dreams. According to Sri Aurobindo such dreams, which Jung ascribed to the collective unconscious, come from the subliminal, described by him as "a greater dream-builder"[14] than the subconscient.

(c) Yet another similarity between the subliminal and the collective unconscious is that just as Sri Aurobindo ascribes the best part of ourselves — our art, poetry, philosophy, etc. — to the influences emanating from the subliminal, so Jung considers the archetypal images of the collective unconscious to represent some of the highest values of the human psyche.

(d) The most significant resemblance between the concepts of the subliminal and the collective unconscious lies in that both are

---

*[6] It is striking that whereas modern psychology has recognized the primary role played by the sexual urge and the urge for power in the motivation of human behaviour, it has overlooked the role of wealth with its associated instinct of greed. By contrast, in Indian psychospiritual thought, greed for wealth is viewed as one of the most powerful motivating forces in human life. Sri Ramakrishna often used the alliterative Bengali phrase *kamini kanchan* (women and gold) to refer to what he regarded as the two strongest lures for a human being.

regarded as "transpersonal" or extending beyond the individual consciousness. However, according to Sri Aurobindo, all parts of the being and corresponding levels of consciousness — physical, vital, mental, subliminal, subconscient and inconscient — are both individual and universal. Therefore, in a sense, the term "collective" is applicable to all parts of the being. But, whereas Jung uses the term "collective" to mean what is common to all mankind, Sri Aurobindo uses the term "universal" to mean what is common to everything in the universe, including the sub-human kingdoms. Furthermore, in his concept of the unconscious, Jung does not distinguish, as Sri Aurobindo does, among what is *below* the conscious (the subconscient), *behind* it (the subliminal) and *above* it (the superconscient). (See footnote *[5].)

Behaviourism — The Second Force

The primary emphasis on unconscious motivation — which is the chief characteristic of depth psychology in general and psychoanalysis in particular — led to a reactionary movement and gave rise to Behaviourism — the Second Force in psychology. The viewpoint of behaviourism was first systematically stated by J.B. Watson in a paper entitled "Psychology as a Behaviorist Views It" published in 1913. Watson stated that the proper subject-matter of psychology is objectively observable behaviour which must be explained as a response to internal and external stimuli. Psychology, said Watson, must become "a purely objective experimental branch of natural science". Deprecating the "mind-gazing" methodology of introspection, and eschewing all hypothetical concepts which cannot be tested experimentally, the new school adopted a purely objective approach based on observation and experiment for the study of behaviour. Using largely rats and other laboratory animals, it sought to explain human behaviour strictly in terms of stimulus and response. Psychology once again became primarily a laboratory science, the old "brass-instrument psychology" being replaced by what some have called a "rat psychology". Behaviourism became the dominant school of psychology in the 1920s, and though its influence has to some extent declined, and though clinical practice has continued to be dominated by psychoanalytical and other non-behaviouristic approaches, behaviourism has to this day occupied a commanding position in the mainstream of academic psychology.

Though diametrically opposed to each other in their views regarding the proper subject-matter of psychology and the appropriate method for studying it, psychoanalysis and behaviourism share one fundamental view in common: they both regard the human being as essentially an animal organism. According to psychoanalysis, the human being, like the animal organism, is driven exclusively by the psychobiological energies of the id; the ego and the superego which, from the psychoanalytic viewpoint, constitute the *sui generis* characteristics of the human being, do not alter the fundamental dynamics attributed to the animal organism, namely, the constant tendency to seek a state of homeostasis or internal equilibrium. According to behaviourism, human behaviour is determined by the same laws of stimulus and response which were discovered by Pavlov in his experiments with dogs and by the same principles of reward and punishment which have been found by Skinner and other neobehaviourists to operate in laboratory animals. Thus both psychoanalysis and behaviourism are characterized by reductionism, which consists in an attempt to explain the complex behaviour of the more highly evolved human organism in terms of the same physiological and biological principles applicable to the simpler behaviour of the less evolved animal organism. Sri Aurobindo made some pertinent observations applicable to this type of reductionism when he wrote:

> ... an ordinary psychology which only takes mind and its phenomena at their surface values, will be of no help to us; it will not give us the least guidance in this line of self-exploration and self-conversion. Still less can we find the clue in a scientific psychology with a materialistic basis which assumes that the

body and the biological and physiological factors of our nature are not only the starting-point but the whole real foundation and regards human mind as only a subtle development from the life and the body. That may be the actual truth of the animal side of human nature and of the human mind in so far as it is limited and conditioned by the physical part of our being. But the whole difference between man and the animal is that the animal mind, as we know it, cannot get for one moment away from its origins, cannot break out from the covering, the close chrysalis which the bodily life has spun round the soul, and become something greater than its present self, a more free, magnificent and noble being; but in man mind reveals itself as a greater energy escaping from the restrictions of the vital and physical formula of being. But even this is not all that man is or can be: he has in him the power to evolve and release a still greater ideal energy which in its turn escapes out of the restrictions of the mental formula of his nature and discloses the supramental form, the ideal power of a spiritual being.[15]

Four Errors of Psychology

Sri Aurobindo pointed out four basic errors afflicting the young science of psychology of his time as evidenced in the major schools of the then psychology reviewed above. He wrote:

It is true that psychology has made an advance and has begun to improve its method. ...The new psychology seeks indeed to penetrate behind superficial appearances, but it is encumbered by initial errors which prevent a profounder knowledge, — the materialistic error which bases the study of mind upon the study of the body; the sceptical error which prevents any bold and clear-eyed investigation of the hidden profundities of our subjective existence; the error of conservative distrust and recoil which regards any subjective state or experience that departs from the ordinary operations of our mental and psychical nature as a morbidity or a hallucination, — just as the Middle Ages regarded all new science as magic and a diabolical departure from the sane and right limits of human capacity; finally, the error of objectivity which leads the psychologist to study others from outside instead of seeing his true field of knowledge and laboratory of experiment in himself. Psychology is necessarily a subjective science and one must proceed in it from the knowledge of oneself to the knowledge of others.[16]

The beginning of efforts for transcending these errors may be discerned in the psychological movements, described below, which took shape subsequently, especially after Sri Aurobindo's passing away in 1950.

Humanistic Psychology — The Third Force

As a reaction to the reductionism of psychoanalysis and behaviourism, there arose what has been called the Third Force in psychology — the school of Humanistic Psychology. According to humanistic psychologists, there are unique aspects of the human being which cannot be adequately explained in terms of the prehuman or animal functioning. One of these unique aspects which is particularly stressed by humanistic psychology is the human individual's inner urge to grow through the development of one's latent potentials. Psychoanalysis regards the human organism as seeking essentially the maintenance of a state of homeostasis. Behaviourism holds that an individual's behaviour is merely a reaction to stimuli. According to humanistic psychology, however, an individual does not seek merely to maintain the existent state of homeostasis, nor can human behaviour be explained solely as response to stimuli: the human being is impelled from within to exceed the actual or existent state in order to actualize the latent potentials. Abraham Maslow (1907-1970), one of the founders of the humanistic movement in psychology, attempted to develop a comprehensive view of human potentials which encompass, in the words of one of the titles of his books, "the farther reaches of human nature", including the attainment of "peak experiences" — states which are generally associated with mystical or semi-mystical experiences. Maslow thus comes close to voicing what has been stated by Sri Aurobindo regarding "the whole difference between man and the animal" in the last but one passage quoted above.

Transpersonal Psychology — The Fourth Force

In turning more and more to the consideration of man's highest potential, Maslow and other humanistic psychologists moved beyond humanism to a consideration of what transcends the ordinary state of human consciousness. During the later phase of his work, Maslow wrote:

> I consider Humanistic, Third Force Psychology, to be transitional, a preparation for a still "higher" Fourth Psychology, transpersonal, transhuman, centered in the cosmos rather than in human needs and interest, going beyond humanness, identity, self-actualization, and the like.[17]

Anthony Sutich (1907-1976), another founder of humanistic psychology, also eventually came to a similar conclusion as Maslow's regarding the humanistic approach. He stated:

> I felt that something was lacking in the [humanistic] orientation... and that it did not ... give sufficient attention to the place of man in the universe or cosmos. A special problem was my growing realization that the concept of self-actualization was no longer comprehensive enough.[18]

The "still 'higher' psychology" envisaged by Maslow strikingly echoes Sri Aurobindo's prevision of "the greater psychology awaiting its hour". In the late 1960s, Maslow, Sutich and other prominent humanistic psychologists founded an association for the study of what they called Transpersonal Psychology, thereby launching the latest major movement in psychology, regarded by a growing number of psychologists as the Fourth Force.

One of the most significant features of transpersonal psychology is the revolutionary view and definition of psychology put forth by some of its votaries. The view has been well expressed by Robert Ornstein who writes:

> Psychology is, primarily, the science of consciousness. Its researchers deal with consciousness directly when possible and indirectly, through the study of physiology and behaviour, when necessary.[19]

Here again we have a partial echo of what Sri Aurobindo had written several decades earlier regarding the nature and scope of psychology. In an unrevised, and perhaps incomplete piece of writing entitled "Psychology", published posthumously, Sri Aurobindo wrote:

> Psychology is the science of consciousness and its states and operations in Nature*[7] and, if that can be glimpsed or experienced, its states and operations beyond what we know as Nature....
>
> Our observable consciousness, that which we call ourselves, is only the little visible part of our being. It is a small field below which are depths and farther depths and widths and ever wider widths which support and supply it but to which it has no visible access. All that is our self, our being, — what we see at the top is only our ego and its visible nature.
>
> Even the movements of this little surface nature cannot be understood nor its true law discovered until we know all that is below or behind and supplies it — and know too all that is around it and above.[20]

*[7] In the experience of yoga, the Self takes two aspects in manifestation, the Purusha (Conscious Being) and Prakriti (Nature). Nature in the individual is his mind, life and body. (Author's note)

It is, of course, not the first time that psychology is being defined as the science of consciousness. It was so defined by E.B. Titchener and other psychologists of the introspectionist school for whom, as previously stated, psychology was the study of the "elements of consciousness". However, what the early introspectionist psychologists studied was the superficial aspect of consciousness, observable through introspection. The study of consciousness did not include what lies outside conscious awareness and what is therefore not accessible to introspection. Regarding this ordinary view of consciousness, Sri Aurobindo writes:

> Consciousness is usually identified with mind, but mental consciousness is only the human range which no more exhausts all the possible ranges of consciousness than human sight exhausts all the gradations of colour or human hearing all the gradations of sound — for there is much above or below that is to man invisible and inaudible. So there are ranges of consciousness above and below the human range, with which the normal human has no contact and they seem to it unconscious, — supramental or overmental and submental ranges.[21]

In Sri Aurobindo's definition of psychology as the science of consciousness the term consciousness does not connote merely our surface consciousness, but a reality which, as stated above, has various ranges, similar to the gradations of colour or of sound. Perhaps the clearest expression of this new concept of consciousness in modern psychology is to be found in Ken Wilber who, using a metaphor similar to those used by Sri Aurobindo in the passage just quoted, has formulated the concept of "the spectrum of consciousness" which he explains as follows:

> ... human personality is a multi-leveled manifestation or expression of a single consciousness, just as in physics the electro-magnetic spectrum is viewed as a multi-banded expression of a single, characteristic electro-magnetic

wave.... Each level of the spectrum is marked by a different and easily recognized sense of individual identity, which ranges from the supreme identity of cosmic consciousness through several gradations or bands to the drastically narrowed sense of identity associated with egoic consciousness.[22]

Wilber's view of ego-consciousness as representing a "drastically narrowed sense of identity" is in some respects a total reversal of what modern psychology has hitherto held regarding the ego. For, from the viewpoint of modern psychology in general and of psychoanalysis in particular, the ego represents the most advanced stage in the psychological development of an individual. A normal and psychologically healthy person is deemed to be one who has an adequately developed ego. When the ego is ill-developed in an individual and, as a result, the individual suffers from certain ego-deficits, or, when after having developed an adequately strong ego there is a breakdown in some of the ego functions due to outer stress or inner conflict, the individual suffers from neurosis or psychosis. Therefore, modern psychology, which has hitherto been preoccupied with what is regarded as the "normal" personality, has extolled the ego, equating a well-developed ego with the state of normality and psychological health. Even Jung, who was strongly influenced by Eastern thought, and who, in his concept of the collective unconscious, was one of the earliest thinkers in modern psychology to speak of something that is transpersonal, did not admit of a state of consciousness in which the ego is transcended or abolished. He categorically asserted that "consciousness is inconceivable without an ego.... If there is no ego there is nobody to be conscious of anything."[23] According to Jung, to lose the ego is to fall into a state of unconsciousness.

The difficulty in conceiving of consciousness without an ego is rooted in the very nature of the normal human consciousness which is ego-bound. But yogic experience testifies that the ego, with its sense of a separate individuality, is only a shadow of the true individuality. The true individuality, says Sri Aurobindo, is characterized by a sense of oneness with the all. As he states: "Our ego is only a face of the universal being and has no separate existence; our apparent separative individuality is only a surface movement and behind it our real individuality stretches out to unity with all things...."[24]

The model of the spectrum of consciousness, which admits of levels of consciousness other than that of the ego, is, according to Wilber, a core concept of the "perennial psychology" — a universal doctrine regarding the nature of man common to all major metapsychological traditions of the world — and "yet at the same time gives ample consideration to the insights of such typical Western disciplines as ego-psychology, psychoanalysis, humanistic psychology, Jungian analysis, interpersonal psychology, and the like."[25]

If psychology is the study of consciousness, the view that consciousness consists of gradations above and below our normal state of ego-consciousness would suggest that the study of psychology and knowledge of the self are intimately related and must go had in hand. This thought has been well expressed by John Welwood. Suggesting the directions that a new psychology might take, Welwood writes:

> This new approach needs to be a *self-knowledge psychology*, based on an inner empiricism, an investigation of experience and its deeper nature....*8
>
> It needs to be based on self-knowledge *disciplines* (such as the practice of meditation). Every body of knowledge is based on a certain discipline, an orderly and precise approach of observing, practising, and learning. A self-knowledge discipline is one in which attention is trained to actively examine the nature of one's experience....[26]

Such a view of psychology as a self-knowledge discipline was

---

*8 The reader may recall what Sri Aurobindo said in speaking about the four basic errors of psychology: "Psychology is necessarily a subjective science and one must proceed in it from the knowledge of oneself to the knowledge of others."

adumbrated by Sri Aurobindo who spoke of "psychological methods of discipline by which man purifies and perfects himself, — the work of psychology, not as it is understood in Europe, but the deeper practical psychology called in India yoga".[27] "Yoga", he said, "is nothing but practical psychology."[28]

In presaging the emergence of psychology as a science of consciousness and as a self-knowledge discipline lies perhaps Sri Aurobindo's greatest relevance to modern psychology. However, besides foreshadowing the "greater psychology awaiting its hour", Sri Aurobindo has through personal exploration and experience mapped out and intimately described a vast terrain of consciousness in its various gradations. Embodied in his yoga, such a science of consciousness, which is also a discipline for attaining self-knowledge, awaits discovery by those who are turning towards the new horizons in psychology.

REFERENCES

1. Sri Aurobindo, *The Human Cycle*, Sri Aurobindo Birth Centenary Library (hereafter SABCL) (Pondicherry: Sri Aurobindo Ashram, 1970-75), Vol. 15, p. 1.
2. Sri Aurobindo, "The Inconscient" in *The Supramental Manifestation and Other Writings*, SABCL, Vol. 16, p. 258.
3. Sri Aurobindo, *Letters on Yoga*, SABCL, Vol. 22, p. 321.
4. Sri Aurobindo, "The Inconscient" in *The Supramental Manifestation and Other Writings*, SABCL, Vol. 16, p. 258.
5. Sri Aurobindo, *Letters on Yoga*, SABCL, Vol. 22, p. 353.
6. Sri Aurobindo, *Letters on Yoga*, SABCL, Vol. 24, p. 1606.
7. *Ibid.*, pp. 1608-09.
8. *Ibid.*, pp. 1297-98.
9. *Ibid.*, pp. 1605-07.
10. Sri Aurobindo, *Letters on Yoga*, SABCL, Vol. 22, p. 321.
11. Sri Aurobindo, *The Mother*, SABCL, Vol. 25, p. 11.
12. Sri Aurobindo, *The Life Divine*, SABCL, Vol. 18, p. 427.
13. C.G. Jung, *Memories, Dreams, Reflections* (London: Routledge and Kegan Paul, 1963), p. 201.
14. Sri Aurobindo, *The Life Divine*, SABCL, Vol. 18, p. 424.

15. Sri Aurobindo, *The Synthesis of Yoga*, SABCL, Vol. 21, pp. 597-98.
16. Sri Aurobindo, "The Inconscient" in *The Supramental Manifestation and Other Writings*, SABCL, Vol. 16. p. 258.
17. Maslow, A. H., *Toward a Psychology of Being* (New York: Van Nostrand Reinhold, 1968).
18. Cited in John Welwood (Ed.), *The Meeting of the Ways* (New York: Shocken Books, 1979), p. 224.
19. Ornstein, R.., *The Psychology of Consciousness* (San Francisco: W.H. Freeman, 1972).
20. Sri Aurobindo, "Psychology" in *The Hour of God and Other Writings*, SABCL, Vol. 17, pp. 21-22.
21. Sri Aurobindo, *Letters on Yoga*, SABCL, Vol. 22, p. 234.
22. Ken Wilber, "*Psychologia Perennis*: The Spectrum of Consciousness", *Journal of Transpersonal Psychology*, 1975, Vol. 7, p. 105.
23. Cited in Swami Ajaya, *Psychotherapy East and West* (Honesdale, Pennsylvania: The Himalayan International Institute, 1983), p. 137.
24. Sri Aurobindo, *The Life Divine*, SABCL, Vol. 18, p. 401.
25. Ken Wilber, *op. cit.*
26. John Welwood (Ed.), *The Meeting of the Ways*, pp. 224-25.
27. Sri Aurobindo, "Our Ideal" in *The Supramental Manifestation and Other Writings*, SABCL, Vol. 16, p. 314.
28. Sri Aurobindo, *The Synthesis of Yoga*, SABCL, Vol. 20, p. 39.

2 SRI AUROBINDO AND THE CONCEPT OF THE UNCONSCIOUS IN PSYCHOLOGY

We are not only what we know of ourselves but an immense more which we do not know; our momentary personality is only a bubble on the ocean of our existence.[1]

SRI AUROBINDO

Our mind and ego are like the crown and dome of a temple jutting out from the waves while the great body of the building is submerged under the surface of the waters.[2]

SRI AUROBINDO

As a metaphysical concept, the unconscious had been spoken of by several European thinkers, including the eminent philosophers Leibnitz and Kant. The first elaborate metaphysical theory of the unconscious was developed by Eduard Von Hartmann in *Philosophie des Unbewussten* (Philosophy of the Unconscious) published in 1869, according to which there is an intelligent, purposive, unconscious will which directs the universe. However, as a psychological construct used for the understanding of human behaviour, the concept of the unconscious is associated with two of the foremost personality theorists, namely, Sigmund Freud and Carl Jung.

Freud, who announced his discovery of the unconscious in 1885, described it as a domain of the mind containing desires, feelings, memories and images which have been repressed because they are too anxiety-provoking to be admitted into consciousness. Though these repressed contents of the unconscious are not accessible to conscious awareness, they play a powerful dynamic role in human behaviour, especially in its psychopathological or abnormal manifestations. To express the enormity of the unconscious as compared to the conscious mind, Freud used the well-known metaphor which depicts the mind as an iceberg, nine-tenths of which — the unconscious — lie hidden beneath the surface of the waters. William

James hailed this discovery in 1901 as "the most important step forward that has occurred in psychology since I have been a student of that science".[3] Though the influence of Freud's theory of the human personality has considerably waned since its heyday, his concept of the unconscious still continues to permeate psychological thought to a wide extent. As a present-day psychologist, John Welwood, observes:

> The unconscious is perhaps the most powerful concept in all of modern psychology. The significance of a broad range of human behavior and experience that had been difficult to explain before Freud, such as dreams, neurotic symptoms, symbolic visions, selective forgetting, slips of the tongue, is now widely recognized, thanks to the explanatory power of the concept of the unconscious.[4]

Sigmund Freud

Freud arrived at the twin concepts of the unconscious and repression as a result of his early experience in treating patients with the "cathartic" method — consisting in the revival of painful repressed memories while in a state of hypnosis — which his older colleague, Joseph Breuer, had been using successfully with hysterical patients. Freud observed that among the painful forgotten memories, those of unacceptable wishes were predominant. He attributed such forgetting to the process of repression by which, according to him, the painful memories are pushed into the depths of the unconscious. Such forgetting through repression is distinguished from ordinary forgetting in that the former makes the forgotten material inaccessible to the conscious mind, whereas things which are forgotten ordinarily can be recalled as they lie in abeyance in what Freud called the preconscious layer of the mind. Thus Freud formulated his topographical theory which divided the mind into three layers — the conscious, the preconscious and the unconscious.

Subsequently, Freud developed his structural theory of personality which conceives of the mental apparatus as made up of three components — the id, consisting of the primitive instinctual energies; the ego, constituted by the thinking part of the mind which exercises cognitive functions such as perception, memory, problem-solving, etc., and the superego which acts as a conscience for the ego in censoring the instinctual demands of the id. In relating the concepts of the earlier topographical theory to his later structural view of personality, Freud stated that whereas the id is the true unconscious, "it is certain that much of the ego is itself unconscious",[5] and the superego too is largely unconscious. Thus, according to Freud, all the three components of what in psychology is vaguely termed mind or psyche form part of the unconscious in varying degrees.

Carl G. Jung

In 1912, Jung presented a more complex view of the unconscious in his work entitled *Psychology of the Unconscious*. He distinguished between the personal unconscious — which, he said, was what Freud spoke about — and the collective unconscious which was Jung's own great discovery. The personal unconscious, according to Jung, is made up not only of repressed painful memories — as Freud originally believed — but also of long-forgotten events, of subliminal perceptions which are below the sensory threshold, and of "everything psychic that has not reached the threshold of consciousness or whose energy-charge is not sufficient to maintain it in consciousness or that will reach consciousness only in the future."[6] Thus with regard to forgotten events he states: "When a thing is forgotten... it simply means that the memory has become subliminal. Its energy has sunk so low that it can no longer appear in consciousness."[7] On the other hand, the collective unconscious, said Jung, consists of basic universal human urges or instincts, and is also the "deposit of ancestral experiences accumulated over millions of years"[8] which have established certain deep psychic predispositions in mankind as a whole. These inherited unconscious predispositions find conscious representation in various potent primordial images called archetypes. According to Jung, archetypes can be found in myths and fairy tales all over the world, and emerge in dreams, fantasies and even in the delusions of the psychotic.

Some of the chief archetypes are those of the Mother, Father, Child, Woman, Man, the Great Mother, the Earth Mother, Mother Nature, God, Demon, the Old Wise Man, Birth, Death, Rebirth, Magic, Unity, the Self and the Circle. Thus, according to Jung, instincts and archetypes are the two chief types of contents which constitute the unconscious. Instincts which are for the preservation and propagation of life, are likened to a stream of psychic energy, the archetypes being the permanent course through which the stream flows. Both instincts and archetypes are of unconscious origin, but operate in the conscious mind — the former as impulses of self-preservation and self-procreation, the latter as universal ideas.

Besides the difference in the nature of their contents, the personal unconscious differs from the collective unconscious in two chief respects. First, the former differs from person to person in the nature of its contents; the latter is the same in all individuals the world over. Secondly, the personal unconscious comes into existence subsequent to the formation of the conscious mind, whereas the collective unconscious antecedes the appearance of the conscious mind.

Freud and Jung — Comparison

There are some similarities as well as differences between Freud's and Jung's views of the unconscious. Chiefly, these consist in the following:

(a) In his earlier topographical theory, Freud looked upon the unconscious as the outcome of repression. Thus he at first held that the unconscious was made up of repressed materials only. Jung, on the other hand, maintained that besides repressions, the personal unconscious contains also long-forgotten memories and subliminal impressions.

(b) In his later structural theory, Freud spoke of the id as the primary stuff out of which the other two structural components of personality — ego and superego — subsequently develop. Since the id is wholly unconscious and consists of instinctual drives, Freud's later concept of the unconscious concurred with Jung's in regarding the unconscious as consisting of instincts as well as what is repressed. However, Jung attributed the repressed memories to the personal unconscious, and regarded the instincts as belonging to the collective unconscious.

(c) The major difference between Freud and Jung regarding the unconscious lies in the distinction made by Jung between the personal and the collective unconscious, and the far greater importance given to the latter.

(d) Freud and Jung differed also in their emphasis on the role of the unconscious in human life. According to Freud's theory, the unconscious plays two main roles. In the first place, being a storehouse of instinctual drives, the unconscious provides the biological energies which motivate all behaviour. Secondly, due to its contents of what has been repressed, it causes various types and degrees of disturbances, ranging from "the psychopathology of everyday life", such as slips of the tongue and selective forgetting, to psychiatric disorders of the various psychoneuroses and psychoses. It is this latter role of the unconscious, related to abnormal and negative aspects of behaviour, that looms large in Freud's theory. All the constructive and creative aspects of behavior were attributed by Freud to the sublimating activities of the conscious ego. On the other hand, Jung, while recognising the role of the unconscious — both personal and collective — in psychopathological behaviour, maintained also that the unconscious is the source of creative ideas and that "archetypal images are among the highest values of the human psyche".[9]

(e) A well-known difference between Freud and Jung pertains to their concepts regarding the nature of the instinctual energies of the unconscious. According to Freud's earlier views, the instinctual energies of the id, which he termed the libido, are essentially sexual. Subsequently, Freud reformulated the concept of instincts and spoke of two classes of instincts — Eros or the life-preservative instincts, including the sexual instinct, and Thanatos or the death instinct. In this later formulation, libido came to be regarded as the energies of Eros, and aggression, turning away from pleasure, etc. as the expression of Thanatos. This subsequent modification of Freud's concept of the instinctual energies never dominated psychoanalytic thinking; the id and its libido have tended to retain their exclusively sexual connotations. On the other hand, Jung, who did not place much emphasis on the role of the sexual impulse, regarded the libido as a general psychic energy which expresses itself in numerous forms, including the sexual urge (Freud), the urge for power (Adler), etc.

Sri Aurobindo

From the viewpoint of Sri Aurobindo, the fundamental limitation of modern psychology in delineating the nature of what it calls the unconscious stems from the mistake of describing the whole of a vast and complex reality in terms of a minuscule part, very much like the groping blind men of the well-known parable who, having each grasped a particular part of an elephant, depicted the whole elephant in terms of the particular part of the elephant's body which he happened to grasp and palpate. Sri Aurobindo has pointed out this error on more than one occasion.[10]

Sri Aurobindo's remark that "you must know the whole before you can know the part"[11] finds elucidation in his description of the various parts of the being given below.

Broadly speaking, Sri Aurobindo distinguishes four elements which make up the totality of man's being: the surface or outer being, the subconscient, the subliminal and the superconscient. In order to understand the nature of this fourfold constitution of the being, certain fundamental views of Sri Aurobindo's philosophy need to be grasped. First, man's being is part of the being of the universe, man being a microcosm of the macrocosm; therefore the psychological nature of man is intimately related to the metaphysical nature of the universe. Secondly, all of the universe is a manifestation of consciousness which has been evolving from the nethermost level — the Inconscient — towards the highest levels of the Superconscient; thus "the emergence and growth of consciousness is the central motive of the evolution and the key to its secret purpose."[12] Thirdly, the evolution of consciousness is preceded by its involution; therefore the Inconscient is a concealed consciousness and "an inverse reproduction of the supreme superconscience"[13]; evolution thus is a process of the return of Inconscience to the supreme Consciousness. Implicit in these fundamental propositions is the view that nothing is truly unconscious or totally devoid of consciousness; therefore the unconscious spoken of in psychology is a misnomer; what is called the unconscious is simply that which lies outside the surface conscious awareness and of which the mind in its ordinary state is not conscious.

In the evolutionary process, the first emergence from the Inconscient is Matter from which the human body is evolved. Regarding the workings of the Inconscient in Matter and the body, Sri Aurobindo states:

> The body... is a creation of the Inconscient and itself inconscient or at least subconscient in parts of itself and much of its hidden action; but what we call the Inconscient is an appearance, a dwelling place, an instrument of a secret Consciousness or a Superconscient which has created the miracle we call the universe. Matter is the field and the creation of the Inconscient and the perfection of the operations of inconscient Matter, their perfect adaptation of means to an aim and end, the wonders they perform and the marvels of beauty they create, testify, in spite of all the ignorant denial we can oppose, to the presence and power of consciousness of this Superconscience in every part and movement of the material universe. It is there in the body, has made it and its emergence in our consciousness is the secret aim of evolution and the key to the mystery of our existence.[14]

From the seemingly inconscient Matter emerge successively Life and Mind. Explaining the nature and function of Life as a middle term between Mind and Matter, Sri Aurobindo writes:

> Life then reveals itself as essentially the same everywhere from the atom to man, the atom containing the subconscious stuff

and movement of being which are released in consciousness in the animal, with plant life as a midway stage in the evolution. Life is really a universal operation of Conscious-Force acting subconsciently on and in Matter; it is the operation that creates, maintains, destroys and re-creates forms or bodies and attempts by play of nerve-force, that is to say, by currents of interchange of stimulating energy to awake conscious sensation in those bodies. In this operation there are three stages; the lowest is that in which the vibration is still in the sleep of Matter, entirely subconscious so as to seem wholly mechanical; the middle stage is that in which it becomes capable of a response still submental but on the verge of what we know as consciousness; the highest is that in which life develops conscious mentality in the form of a mentally perceptible sensation which in this transition becomes the basis for the development of sense-mind and intelligence. It is in the middle stage that we catch the idea of Life as distinguished from Matter and Mind, but in reality it is the same in all the stages and always a middle term between Mind and Matter, constituent of the latter and instinct with the former.[15]

The Surface Being

To return to Sri Aurobindo's fourfold classification of the human constitution, man's surface consciousness, derived from the three universal principles just mentioned, is composed of mind, life (generally referred to by Sri Aurobindo as the vital) and body-consciousness. Sri Aurobindo states that the term "mind", which has been used indiscriminately to cover the whole surface consciousness, connotes in the language of his yoga that part of the being which is related to cognitive elements and functions, such as ideas and thoughts, intelligence, thinking and reasoning. He distinguishes mind from the other two elements of the surface nature, namely, the vital and the body-consciousness, which are mixed up with mind on the surface. The vital is the Life-Nature made up of sensations, energies of action, instincts, impulses, desires, feelings and emotions. The body, says Sri Aurobindo, "is not mere unconscious Matter: it is a structure of a secretly conscious Energy that has taken form in it. Itself occultly conscious, it is, at the same time, the vehicle of expression of an overt Consciousness that has emerged and is self-aware in our physical energy-substance."[16] Regarding the confounding of the vital and the body-consciousness with mind, Sri Aurobindo explains:

> Mind identifies itself to a certain extent with the movements proper to physical life and body and annexes them to its mentality, so that all consciousness seems to us to be mental. But if we draw back, if we separate the mind as witness from these parts of us, we can discover that life and body,— even the most physical parts of life,— have a consciousness of their own, a consciousness proper to an obscurer vital and to a bodily being, even such an elemental awareness as primitive animal forms may have, but in us partly taken up by the mind and to that extent mentalised. Yet it has not, in its independent motion, the mental awareness which we enjoy; if there is mind in it, it is mind involved and implicit in the body and in the physical life: there is no organised self-consciousness, but only a sense of action and reaction, movement, impulse and desire, need, necessary activities imposed by Nature, hunger, instinct, pain, insensibility and pleasure. Although thus inferior, it has this awareness obscure, limited and automatic;... when we stand back from it, when we can separate our mind from its sensations, we perceive that this is a nervous and sensational and automatically dynamic mode of consciousness, a gradation of awareness different from the mind: it has its own separate reactions to contacts and is sensitive to them in its own power of feeling; it does not depend for that on the mind's perception and response.[17]

The Subconscient and the Inconscient
Sri Aurobindo defines the subconscient as follows:

> The subconscious in us is the extreme border of our secret inner existence where it meets the Inconscient, it is a degree of our being in which the Inconscient struggles into a half-

consciousness;... Or, from another viewpoint, this nether part of us may be described as the antechamber of the Inconscient.[18]

An important distinction to be made for understanding the nature of the subconscient is between the submental and the subconscient. The former refers to that which, from the evolutionary point of view, is lower than or inferior to mind. The physical consciousness of the body and that of the vital are in this sense submental, but they are not entirely subconscient, for in them consciousness has already evolved a certain degree of its formulation and expression, though for the most part the operations of consciousness in the physical and vital parts of our being are subconscious to the mind and would therefore be regarded in modern psychology as part of the unconscious. "The true subconscious", says Sri Aurobindo, "is other than this vital or physical substratum; it is the Inconscient vibrating on the borders of consciousness...."[19] In other words, whereas the submental is that which is below mind, the subconscient is what lies below even the physical and body-consciousness.

Sri Aurobindo elaborates the description of the subconscient in the following extracts which reiterate some of its basic characteristics:

> The subconscient is universal as well as individual like all the other main parts of the Nature. But there are different parts or planes of the subconscient. All upon earth is based on the Inconscient as it is called, though it is not really inconscient at all, but rather a complete "sub"-conscience, a suppressed or involved consciousness, in which there is everything but nothing is formulated or expressed. The subconscient lies between this Inconscient and the conscious mind, life and body. It contains the potentiality of all the primitive reactions to life which struggle out to the surface from the dull and inert strands of Matter and form by a constant development a slowly evolving and self-formulating consciousness; it contains them not as ideas, perceptions or conscious reactions but as the fluid substance of these things. But also all that is consciously experienced sinks down into the subconscient, not as precise though

submerged memories but as obscure yet obstinate impressions of experience, and these can come up at any time as dreams, as mechanical repetitions of past thought, feelings, action, etc., as "complexes" exploding into action and event, etc., etc. The subconscient is the main cause why all things repeat themselves and nothing ever gets changed except in appearance. It is the cause why people say character cannot be changed, the cause also of the constant return of things one hoped to have got rid of for ever.[20]

In our yoga we mean by the subconscient that quite submerged part of our being in which there is no wakingly conscious and coherent thought, will or feeling or organized reaction, but which yet receives obscurely the impressions of all things and stores them up in itself and from it too all sorts of stimuli, of persistent habitual movements, crudely repeated or disguised in strange forms can surge up into dream or into the waking nature. For if these impressions rise up most in dream in an incoherent and disorganized manner, they can also and do rise up into our waking consciousness as a mechanical repetition of old thoughts, old mental, vital and physical habits or an obscure stimulus to sensations, actions, emotions which do not originate in or from our conscious thought or will and are even often opposed to its perceptions, choice or dictates. In the subconscient there is an obscure mind full of obstinate Sanskaras, impressions, associations, fixed notions, habitual reactions formed by our past, an obscure vital full of the seeds of habitual desires, sensations and nervous reactions, a most obscure material which governs much that has to do with the condition of the body. It is largely responsible for our illnesses; chronic or repeated illnesses are indeed mainly due to the subconscient and its obstinate memory and habit of repetition of whatever has impressed itself upon the body-consciousness.[21]

It is a known psychological law that whatever is suppressed in the conscious mind remains in the subconscient being and recurs either in the waking state when the control is removed or

Sri Aurobindo and the Concept of the Unconscious

else in sleep. Mental control by itself cannot eradicate anything entirely out of the being. The subconscient in the ordinary man includes the larger part of the vital being and the physical mind and also the secret body-consiousness.[22]

When something is thrown out of the vital or physical, it very usually goes down into the subconscient and remains there as if in seed and comes up again when it can. That is the reason why it is so difficult to get rid of habitual vital movements or to change the character; for, supported or refreshed from this source, preserved in this matrix your vital movements, even when suppressed or repressed, surge up again and recur.[23]

That part of us which we can strictly call subconscient because it is below the level of mind and conscious life, inferior and obscure, covers the purely physical and vital elements of our constitution of bodily being, unmentalised, unobserved by the mind, uncontrolled by it in their action. It can be held to include the dumb occult consciousness, dynamic but not sensed by us, which operates in the cells and nerves and all the corporeal stuff and adjusts their life process and automatic responses. It covers also those lowest functionings of submerged sense-mind which are more operative in the animal and in plant life.[24]

It is interesting to note that some of Freud's basic views regarding the unconscious strikingly reflect the description of the subconscient as given above. The following are among the chief of such Freudian views of the unconscious which are corroborated by Sri Aurobindo in describing the nature of the subconscient:
  (a) The unconscious is far more extensive than the conscious.
  (b) What is repressed or driven out of conscious awareness becomes part of the unconscious.
  (c) The contents of the unconscious powerfully affect the workings of the conscious mind.
  (d) What lies in the unconscious emerges in dreams. (Dreams, said Freud, are the royal road to the unconscious.)
  (e) Certain experiences rooted in the unconscious tend to be

re-enacted repeatedly in a compulsive way — what Freud termed "repetition compulsion".

However, according to Sri Aurobindo, "the lower vital subconscious which is all that this psycho-analysis of Freud seems to know,—and even of that it knows only a few ill-lit corners,—is no more than a restricted and very inferior portion of the subliminal whole.[25]

The Subliminal

The term "subliminal" literally means below the threshold, and in its current usage is generally employed with reference to sensory stimuli which are below the detection threshold, that is, are of less than the minimum intensity or duration required to excite a sensory neuron and be perceived. In 1886, F.W.H. Myers, to whom the discovery of the subliminal is ascribed, used the term to describe certain psychological processes which take place below the level of awareness. Subsequently, in the writings of Jung and others, the term was used at times as a synonym for the unconscious (or the subconscious as it has sometimes been called). Referring to this last-mentioned usage of the term as co-extensive with what in modern psychology has been called the unconscious or the subconscious, Sri Aurobindo states:

> Subliminal is a general term used for all parts of the being which are not on the waking surface. Subconscient is very often used in the same sense by European psychologists because they do not know the difference. But when I use the word [subconscient], I mean always what is below the ordinary physical consciousness, not what is behind it.[26]

Sri Aurobindo has occasionally used "subliminal" as a general term to denote all parts of the being which are not on the waking surface consciousness, "so conceiving it as to include in it our lower subconscient and upper superconscient ends."[27] However, for the most part he distinguishes three parts of the being which are outside the surface consciousness: that which lies below (the subconscient), that which lies behind (the subliminal), and that which is high above

Sri Aurobindo and the Concept of the Unconscious

(the superconscient). Regarding the distinction between the subconscient and the subliminal, Sri Aurobindo states:

> The real subconscious is a nether diminished consciousness close to the Inconscient; the subliminal is a consciousness larger than our surface existence. But both belong to the inner realm of our being of which our surface is unaware, so both are jumbled together in our common conception and parlance.[28]

> ...when we say subconscious, we think readily of an obscure unconsciousness or half-consciousness or else a submerged consciousness below and in a way inferior to and less than our organised waking awareness or, at least, less in possession of itself. But we find, when we go within, that somewhere in our subliminal part, — though not co-extensive with it since it has also obscure and ignorant regions, — there is a consciousness much wider, more luminous, more in possession of itself and things than that which wakes upon our surface and is the percipient of our daily hours; that is our inner being, and it is this which we must regard as our subliminal self and set apart the subconscient as an inferior, a lowest occult province of our nature.[29]

Sri Aurobindo states further the nature of the subliminal self as follows:

> The subliminal self stands behind and supports the whole superficial man; it has in it a larger and more efficient mind behind the surface mind, a larger and more powerful vital behind the surface vital, a subtler and freer physical consciousness behind the surface bodily existence. And above them it opens to higher superconscient as well as below them to lower subconscient ranges.[30]

> There is a "subliminal" self behind our superficial waking mind, not inconscient but conscient, greater than the waking mind, endowed with surprising faculties and capable of a much surer

action and experience, conscient of the superficial mind, though of it the superficial mind is inconscient.[31]

Our subliminal self is not, like our surface physical being, an outcome of the energy of the Inconscient; it is a meeting-place of the consciousness that emerges from below by evolution and the consciousness that has descended from above for involution. There is in it an inner mind, an inner vital being of ourselves, an inner or subtle-physical being larger than our outer being and nature. ... There is here a consciousness which has a power of direct contact with the universal unlike the mostly indirect contacts which our surface being maintains with the universe through the sense-mind and the senses. There are here inner senses, a subliminal sight, touch, hearing; but these subtle senses are rather channels of the inner being's direct consciousness of things than its informants: the subliminal is not dependent on its senses for its knowledge, they only give a form to its direct experience of objects; they do not, so much as in waking mind, convey forms of objects for the mind's documentation or as the starting-point or basis for an indirect constructive experience. The subliminal has the right of entry into the mental and vital and subtle-physical planes of the universal consciousness, it is not confined to the material plane and the physical world; it possesses means of communication with the worlds of being which the descent towards involution created in its passage and with all corresponding planes or worlds that may have arisen or been constructed to serve the purpose of the re-ascent from Inconscience to Superconscience. It is into this large realm of interior existence that our mind and vital being retire when they withdraw from the surface activities whether by sleep or inward-drawn concentration or by the inner plunge of trance.[32]

Sri Aurobindo has called the subliminal self the inner being as distinguished from the outer or surface being. Thus he states:

There are, we might say, two beings in us, one on the surface, our ordinary exterior mind, life, body consciousness, another behind the veil, an inner mind, an inner life, an inner physical consciousness constituting another or inner self.[33]

The outer being is connected with the subliminal and, though unaware of it, receives from the subliminal its inspirations, intuitions, etc. As Sri Aurobindo states:

> It [the subliminal] is, according to our psychology, connected with the small outer personality by certain centres of consciousness of which we become aware by yoga. Only a little of the inner being escapes through these centres into the outer life, but that little is the best part of ourselves and responsible for our art, poetry, philosophy, ideals, religious aspirations, efforts at knowledge and perfection.[34]

Thus though the surface being of the average individual is largely influenced by the subconscient it is also influenced to a significant extent by the subliminal.

Jung's concept of the collective unconscious reflects several aspects of what Sri Aurobindo describes as the subliminal. For example, in the subliminal, as stated above, are inner senses of sight, touch, hearing, etc.; the subliminal is therefore "the seer of inner things and supraphysical experiences."[35] Jung, who reports having had frequent supraphysical experiences such as visions or what he called "extremely vivid hypnagogic images",[36] ascribed such experiences to the collective unconscious. Another striking resemblance between Sri Aurobindo's description of the subliminal and Jung's view of the collective unconscious lies in tracing the source of predictive, veridical and deeply symbolic dreams. According to Sri Aurobindo such dreams, which Jung ascribed to the collective unconscious, come from the subliminal, which he described as "a greater dream-builder"[37] than the subconscient. Yet another similarity between the subliminal and the collective unconscious is that just as Sri Aurobindo ascribes the best part of ourselves — our art, poetry, philosophy, etc. — to the influences emanating from the subliminal, so Jung, as stated earlier, considers the archetypal images of the collective unconscious to be some of the highest values of the human psyche. The most significant resemblance between the concepts of the subliminal and the collective unconscious lies in that both are regarded as "transpersonal" or extending beyond the individual consciousness. However, according to Sri Aurobindo, all parts of the being or levels of consciousness mentioned above — physical, vital, mental, subconscient, inconscient and subliminal — are both individual and universal. Therefore, in a sense, the term "collective" is applicable to all parts of the being. Moreover, whereas Jung uses the term "collective" to mean what is common to all mankind, Sri Aurobindo uses the term "universal" to mean what is common to everything in the universe, including the sub-human kingdoms. Furthermore, in his concept of the unconscious, Jung does not distinguish, as Sri Aurobindo does, among what is below (subconscient), behind (subliminal) and above (superconscient) in relation to the surface consciousness.

The Superconscient

As stated previously, the superconscient is the starting point of the involution of consciousness and the ultimate goal of its evolution. Regarding the superconscient, Sri Aurobindo writes:

> If the subliminal and subconscient may be compared to a sea which throws up the waves of our surface mental existence, the superconscience may be compared to an ether which constitutes, contains, overroofs, inhabits and determines the movements of the sea and its waves. It is there in this higher ether that we are inherently and intrinsically conscious of our self and spirit, not as here below by a reflection in silent mind or by acquisition of the knowledge of a hidden Being within us; it is through it, through that ether of superconscience, that we can pass to a supreme status, knowledge, experience. Of this superconscient existence through which we can arrive at the highest status of our real, our supreme Self, we are normally even more ignorant than of the rest of our being; yet is it into the knowledge of it that our being emerging out of the involu-

tion in Inconscience is struggling to evolve.[38]

In the superconscience beyond our present level of awareness are included the higher planes of mental being as well as the native heights of supramental and pure spiritual being.[39]

Among the higher planes of mental being, Sri Aurobindo distinguishes various distinct levels which he terms Higher Mind, Illumined Mind, Intuitive Mind and Overmind, culminating in what Sri Aurobindo calls Supermind or the Truth-Consciousness which secretly supports all the universe and leads all towards itself through the evolutionary process. There seems to be little in Jung's concept of the collective unconscious that reflects these planes of the superconscient.

Knowing the Unconscious

In the last chapter ("Late Thoughts") of his *Memories, Dreams, Reflections*, Jung points out the inability of the mind to know the unconscious. He writes:

> Science employs the term 'the unconscious', thus admitting that it knows nothing about it, for it can know nothing about the substance of the psyche when the sole means of knowing anything is the psyche.[40]

Sri Aurobindo goes a step further and points out that the mind, because of its inherent limitations, is incapable of knowing *anything* in its essential nature. As he states:

> Mind in its essence is a consciousness which measures, limits, cuts out forms of things from the indivisible whole and contains them as if each were a separate integer.[41]

> Mind is an instrument of analysis and synthesis, but not of essential knowledge. Its function is to cut out something vaguely from the unknown thing in itself and call this measurement or

delimitation of it the whole, and again to analyse the whole into its parts which it regards as separate mental objects.[42]

Because of the intrinsic limitations of the mind as stated above, the method employed for understanding the unconscious, consisting in a mental analysis of what are believed to be the products of the unconscious, namely, dreams, free-associations, etc., has yielded only fragmentary and relatively superficial insights into the so-called unconscious. From these limited insights the mind has sought to construct the total reality of that which lies below, behind and beyond mind. As a result, the whole has either been reduced and explained in terms of a fragment, as in Freud's concept of the unconscious, or subsumed under a nebulous and conglomerate concept such as Jung's collective unconscious. The latest major school of psychological thought — Transpersonal Psychology — has come to recognise a wider range of phenomena, experiences and states of consciousness which have hitherto been regarded by most psychologists as belonging to a "fringe" area, such as extrasensory perception, telepathy, precognition, telekinesis, clairvoyance and clairaudience, "peak" experiences, altered states of consciousness, etc. which are now classed under the ill-defined concept of "transpersonal consciousness", the heterogeneous nature of which may be seen from the following statement:

> Transpersonal content includes any experiences in which an individual transcends the limitations of identifying exclusively with the ego or personality. Transpersonal content also includes the mythical, archetypal, and symbolic realms of inner experience that can come into awareness through imagery and dreams.[43]

According to Sri Aurobindo, in order to know what lies outside mental awareness and be able to distinguish among the subconscient, the subliminal and the superconscient, it is necessary to break the walls that separate the surface consciousness from what lies behind and beyond it so as to emerge into the subliminal and the superconscient. As he states:

A descent into the subconscient would not help us to explore this region, for it would plunge us into incoherence or into sleep or a dull trance or a comatose torpor. A mental scrutiny or insight can give us some indirect and constructive idea of these hidden activities; but it is only by drawing back into the subliminal or by ascending into the superconscient and from there looking down or extending ourselves into these obscure depths that we can become directly and totally aware and in control of the secrets of our subconscient physical, vital and mental nature.[44]

...though large parts of it [the subliminal] can be thus known by a penetration and looking within or a freer communication, it is only by going inward behind the veil of superficial mind and living within, in an inner mind, an inner life, an inmost soul of our being that we can be fully self-aware,— by this and by rising to a higher plane of mind than that which our waking consciousness inhabits. An enlargement and completion of our present evolutionary status, now still so hampered and truncated, would be the result of such an inward living; but an evolution beyond it can come only by our becoming conscious in what is now superconscient to us, by an ascension to the native heights of the Spirit.[45]

Conclusion

From Sri Aurobindo's viewpoint, no part of the being is devoid of consciousness. Therefore the term "unconscious" is a misnomer. What is called the unconscious in Western psychology is simply that which lies outside the surface mental consciousness and of which the *mind in its ordinary state is unconscious.*

Broadly speaking, Sri Aurobindo distinguishes three levels of consciousness which lie outside mental awareness: the subconscient, a *nether* level of consciousness below the surface nature; the subliminal, a *deeper* level of consciousness behind the frontal being; and the superconscient, a *higher* level of consciousness above the surface being. In Western psychology, all the three have been indiscriminately referred to as "the unconscious".

The description of the unconscious given by Freud has a number of characteristics of what Sri Aurobindo has termed the subconscient. Freud's concept of the unconscious does not reflect any elements of what Sri Aurobindo speaks of as the subliminal and the superconscient. Therefore, in Freud's thought, everything that lies outside normal awareness is reduced to what he called the unconscious.

Jung's concept of the collective unconscious reflects several elements which Sri Aurobindo ascribes to the subliminal. But Jung does not distinguish among what Sri Aurobindo calls the subconscient, the subliminal and the superconscient, to all of which the term "collective" — in the sense of what exceeds individual limits — is equally applicable.

REFERENCES

1. Sri Aurobindo, *The Life Divine*, Sri Aurobindo Birth Centenary Library (hereafter SABCL) (Pondicherry: Sri Aurobindo Ashram, 1970-75), Vol. 18, p. 555.
2. Ibid., p. 556.
3. William James, *The Varieties of Religious Experience*. New York: Longman, Green & Co., 1928, p. 233.
4. John Welwood (Ed.), *The Meeting of the Ways*. New York: Schocken Books, 1979, p. 151.
5. Cited in Roger N. Walsh and Frances Vaughan (Eds.) *Beyond Ego: Transpersonal Dimensions in Psychology*. Los Angeles: Jeremy P. Tarcher, 1980, p. 109.
6. C. G. Jung, *The Collected Works of C.G. Jung*. Translated by R.F.C. Hull. Bollingen Series XX, Vol. X. New York: Pantheon Books, 1964, p. 8.
7. Ibid.
8. C. G. Jung, *The Collected Works of C.G. Jung*, Vol. VIII, p. 376.
9. C. G. Jung, *The Collected Works of C.G. Jung*, Vol. IX, Part I, p. 84.
10. Vide references 3 and 14 of the essay on "Sri Aurobindo and Modern Psychology".
11. Sri Aurobindo, *Letters on Yoga*, SABCL, Vol. 24, p. 1609.
12. Sri Aurobindo, *The Supramental Manifestation and Other Writings*, SABCL, Vol. 16, p. 16.

13. Sri Aurobindo, *The Life Divine*, SABCL, Vol. 18, p. 550.
14. Sri Aurobindo, *The Supramental Manifestation and Other Writings*, SABCL, Vol. 16, pp. 10-11.
15. Sri Aurobindo, *The Life Divine*, SABCL, Vol. 18, p. 186.
16. Ibid., p. 305.
17. Ibid., pp. 558-59.
18. Ibid., pp. 422-23.
19. Ibid., p. 559.
20. Sri Aurobindo, *Letters on Yoga*, SABCL, Vol. 22, pp. 354-55.
21. Ibid., p. 353.
22. Sri Aurobindo, *Letters on Yoga*, SABCL, Vol. 23, p. 898.
23. Sri Aurobindo, *Letters on Yoga*, SABCL, Vol. 22, p. 357.
24. Sri Aurobindo, *The Life Divine*, SABCL, Vol. 19, pp. 733-34.
25. Sri Aurobindo, *Letters on Yoga*, SABCL, Vol. 24, p. 1606.
26. Sri Aurobindo, *Letters on Yoga*, SABCL, Vol. 22, p. 354.
27. Sri Aurobindo, *The Life Divine*, SABCL, Vol. 18, p. 557.
28. Ibid., p. 223fn.
29. Ibid., p. 557.
30. Sri Aurobindo, *Letters on Yoga*, SABCL, Vol. 24, p. 1606.
31. Sri Aurobindo, *The Supramental Manifestation and Other Writings*, SABCL, Vol. 16, p. 261.
32. Sri Aurobindo, *The Life Divine*, SABCL, Vol. 18, pp. 425-26.
33. Sri Aurobindo, *Letters on Yoga*, SABCL, Vol. 23, pp. 1020-21.
34. Sri Aurobindo, *Letters on Yoga*, SABCL, Vol. 24, pp. 1164-65.
35. Sri Aurobindo, *The Life Divine*, SABCL, Vol. 18, p. 427.
36. C.G. Jung, *Memories, Dreams, Reflections*. London: Routledge and Kegan Paul, 1963, p. 201.
37. Sri Aurobindo, *The Life Divine*, SABCL, Vol. 18, p. 424.
38. Ibid., pp. 561-62.
39. Sri Aurobindo, *The Life Divine*, SABCL, Vol. 19, p. 736.
40. C.G. Jung, *Memories, Dreams, Reflections*, p. 310.
41. Sri Aurobindo, *The Life Divine*, SABCL, Vol. 18, p. 162.
42. Ibid., p. 127.
43. Frances Vaughan, "Transpersonal Psychotherapy: Context, Content, and Process" in *Beyond Ego: Transpersonal Dimensions in Psychology*, p. 185.
44. Sri Aurobindo, *The Life Divine*, SABCL, Vol. 19, p. 734.
45. Ibid., p. 736.

3 SELF-AWARENESS IN PSYCHOLOGY AND SRI AUROBINDO'S YOGA

The well-known present-day physicist, Fritjof Capra, has pointed out the emerging concurrence between modern physics and the ancient spiritual wisdom in their views regarding the nature of the universe.[1] In the field of modern psychology, too, especially in one of its latest schools — Transpersonal Psychology — one can discern the beginnings of a concurrence, though as yet quite rudimentary, between scientific psychology and spirituality, not only in their theoretical views regarding the nature of the human being but also in their practical approaches for the attainment of growth and well-being. The present essay is an attempt to study from the perspective of Sri Aurobindo's Yoga one of the pivotal topics which serves to bring out parallels as well as differences between modern psychology and yoga.

At a symposium on "Consciousness" held in 1977 at the California Institute of Transpersonal Psychology, one of the speakers observed that there has been in the United States a growing cult of "awareness", even though most people who use the slogan of awareness do not quite seem to know what they want to become aware of.

Some of the earliest beginnings of the wide interest presently prevailing in the West in the development of awareness may be traced to the movement of psychoanalysis which, until relatively recently, held most sway in the field of mental health. According to psychoanalysis, human behaviour, especially in its more abnormal and pathological forms, is predominantly determined by elements of personality of which the individual is unconscious. The principal aim of the psychoanalytic procedure, therefore, is to impart insight into the unconscious dynamics of one's behaviour. According to the psychoanalytic theory, such insight into the unconscious origins and motivations of one's behaviour brings about therapeutic changes by enthroning the rational and more conscious part of the personality, namely, the Ego, in place of the irrational, unconscious, instinctive drives of the Id, and the equally unconscious parental introjections of the Super-ego. Thus what is called insight in psychoanalysis is an awareness of the unconscious psychodynamics underlying one's personality make-up and behaviour.

Carl Jung, who broke away from psychoanalysis, held that besides the personal unconscious which is specific to each individual, there is another greater layer of the unconscious — the collective unconscious — which is common to the human race as a whole. The collective unconscious, according to Jung, contains what he calls archetypes or universal "complexes of experience" which are at the basis of all behaviour, both instinctive and acquired, and which play a far greater role in moulding an individual's life than the personal unconscious which psychoanalysis deals with. Jung cites the example of a person whose neurosis persisted even after gaining insight into his personal unconscious through years of psychoanalysis; it was only after acquiring insight into the specific archetype underlying his neurotic behaviour that he was able to overcome his neurosis. As long as one is unconscious of the archetype governing a certain form of behaviour, one does not act as an individual but as a blind tool of a collective force. The aim of Jungian analysis is to bring about individuation by making one conscious of the archetypes governing one's life and freeing one from bondage to their dictates. Thus Jung's Analytical Psychology concerns itself essentially with the development of awareness pertaining to the collective unconscious and its archetypes in their influence on one's behaviour.

Alfred Adler, who, too, abandoned psychoanalysis, believed that neurotic behaviour can be explained more satisfactorily in terms of an urge for power rather than the drive for pleasure as postulated by Freud. According to Adler, neurosis is due to an inferiority complex arising out of a real or imagined inferiority in respect of one or more characteristics pertaining to one's physique, intelligence, psychological traits, socio-economic status, ethnicity, etc. The neurotic person unconsciously "arranges" his symptoms so as to compensate for the feelings of inferiority. As a result, different kinds of neurotic behaviour ensue, such as displaying a sense of superiority, a compulsive need to compete and win against others, an inordinate aggressiveness, etc. or their very opposites, namely, a feeling of inferiority, a fear of competition and achievement, passivity, etc. As a reaction to the Freudian over-emphasis on the analysis of the unconscious, Adlerian psychotherapy adopts an educational approach which focuses on helping the neurotic individual to learn healthy and constructive ways of overcoming the inferiority complex. Thus the aim in Adler's approach is education rather than insight. However, in interpreting the patient's symptoms in terms of an unconscious inferiority complex, and explaining his behaviour as an unconscious attempt to compensate for the feeling of inferiority so as to attain a fictitious sense of power, Adlerian psychotherapy does lead the patient to a greater awareness of himself by giving him an insight into the unconscious underpinnings of his personality and behaviour.

Gestalt Therapy, also an outgrowth of psychoanalysis, avowedly regards the development of awareness as the very essence of the therapeutic process. For, according to Gestalt Therapy, the neurotic individual characteristically suffers from a lack of adequate awareness, especially of his feelings and of the here and now. Thus the neurotic person may be angry at someone and may express his anger indirectly through behaviour without being aware of his feelings of anger. Again, when going through an experience, the neurotic has an inadequate emotional and cognitive contact with what is transpiring in the here and now, and therefore lacks an adequate awareness of what he is experiencing at any given moment. The fundamental process of Gestalt Therapy, therefore, consists in the training of awareness by means of various exercises, experiments and other techniques.

Transactional Analysis, originated by Eric Berne, one of Freud's pupils, views the human personality as consisting of three basic aspects — Child, Adult and Parent, corresponding to Freud's Id, Ego and Super-ego. Berne maintains that the Freudian concepts just mentioned are hypothetical constructs for interpreting human behaviour, whereas Child, Adult and Parent are "phenomenological realities", that is, actual psychological states which can be observed through a person's speech, tone of voice, body gestures and facial expressions. However, though the three psychological states are observable, not many have an insight into their psychological states or the ways in which a particular psychological state influences and is expressed through their behaviour at any given moment. Transactional Analysis seeks to impart such an insight through an analysis of an individual's "transactions" or social interactions. Thus the aim of Transactional Analysis is to bring about therapeutic or growth-inducing changes in the personality by promoting the individual's self-understanding and self-awareness pertaining to the psychological states of Child, Adult and Parent as they determine behaviour; the goal is to have, in Berne's words, "the adult ego maintain hegemony over the impulsive child". Besides the awareness of the three basic psychological states, Transactional Analysis also seeks to inculcate an awareness of the various "scripts" or ingrained patterns of behaviour which develop in childhood and continue inappropriately in adulthood.

It will be seen from what has been stated thus far that though systems of psychotherapy which were developed subsequent to the depth psychologies of Freud and Jung abandoned the concept of the unconscious, and shifted the emphasis from inculcation of insight to change of behaviour, they nevertheless involve, in some measure, the development of insight and the enhancement of awareness pertaining to aspects of personality and behaviour of which the individual is more or less unconscious.

Such a trend is exemplified also in the non-analytical system of Rational-Emotive Therapy (RET) formulated by Albert Ellis. According to RET, psychological disturbances are generally the result of certain fallacies implicit in an individual's beliefs and attitudes. Ellis explains what he calls the A-B-C-D theory of RET as follows. An Activating event of experience (A) seems to cause a certain psychologically disturbing Consequence (C) in an individual. But on closer examination, it will be found that A does not in fact cause C. What causes C is a certain Belief (B) of the individual. For instance, when a person is emotionally upset because someone does not like him or is critical of him, the real cause of the person's emotional disturbance, according to Ellis, lies in his implicit fallacious belief and attitude that we must be liked by everyone and that everyone must approve of everything we do. Ellis, who has identified twelve of the most prevalent fallacious beliefs and attitudes underlying emotional disturbances, maintains that the solution to the problem lies in successfully learning to Dispute (D) one's irrational beliefs. As he states: "RET vigorously helps people to confront and attack their disturbance-creating beliefs. It clearly brings their magical (Illogical and/or self-defeating) philosophies to their attention, explains how these cause emotional upset, attacks them on logico-empirical grounds, and teaches people how to change disordered thinking."[2] Though the major part of the RET process consists in teaching people how to "dispute" their false beliefs, the first step, as implied in Ellis's statements, is to bring their fallacious beliefs "to their attention", that is, to increase their awareness of the beliefs and attitudes underlying their emotional reactions.

Quite unlike the aforementioned systems of therapy is Roberto Assagioli's system of Psychosynthesis. The focus of Psychosynthesis, as its name implies, is, not analysis, but a synthesis of the various conflicting parts of the personality — called sub-personalities — by bringing them to function more and more in harmony with one another and in subordination to what is regarded as the core of the personality, namely, the Self. Though Psychosynthesis is avowedly anti-analytical, its methods, like those of the analytical and non-analytical systems, lead to a greater awareness of aspects of personality of which an individual is largely unconscious. Thus by means of various techniques, such as visualisation, guided imagery, etc., Psychosynthesis seeks to make a person aware of the multiple parts which make up the personality with a view to enabling the person to synthesize and harmonize them.

The preceding brief survey of some of the chief systems of therapy and personal growth is meant to show that despite differences in their theories regarding the structure of personality, the dynamics of behaviour and the methods for bringing about positive psychological changes, they share in common one fundamental element, namely, the inculcation of a greater awareness of aspects of personality and behaviour of which an individual is more or less unaware.

*

Self-Awareness

Those who are well familiar with Sri Aurobindo's Yoga cannot fail to be impressed with the parallels between some of the above-stated views of psychotherapy and the teachings of his Integral Yoga regarding the fact that there are many parts or aspects of oneself of which the individual is largely unaware and of which one needs to be conscious for achieving inner harmony. The basic teachings of Integral Yoga in this regard are expressed in the following two quotations from Sri Aurobindo and the Mother respectively:

> Men do not know themselves and have not learned to distinguish the different parts of their being; for these are usually lumped together by them as mind, because it is through a mentalised perception and understanding that they know or feel them; therefore they do not understand their own states and actions, or, if at all, then only on the surface. It is part of the foundation of yoga to become conscious of the great complexity of our nature, see the different forces that move it and get over it a control of directing knowledge.[3]

> To work for your perfection, the first step is to become conscious of yourself, of the different parts of your being and their respective activities. You must learn to distinguish these different parts one from another, so that you may become clearly aware of the origin of the movements that occur in you, the many impulses, reactions and conflicting wills that drive you to action.[4]

It has been found, especially in psychoanalysis, that sometimes a genuine insight into the unconscious dynamics of one's psychological disturbance has in itself a powerful therapeutic effect. Such a finding, too, has its parallel in yoga. As Sri Aurobindo states:

> ...knowledge, when it goes to the root of our troubles, has in itself a marvellous healing-power as it were. As soon as you touch the quick of the trouble, as soon as you, diving down and down, get at what really ails you, the pain disappears as though by a miracle.[5]

But perhaps the most significant parallelism which seems to be emerging between psychology and yoga lies in the concept of consciousness. During the early phase of its development as a science, psychology was defined as the science of consciousness, and, a little later, as the science of the mind. But the concepts of consciousness and mind were subsequently abandoned as vague and unscientific, and are eschewed by the great majority of present-day psychologists who define psychology as the science of behaviour. However, various developments in the field of psychology have in recent years revived an interest in the study of consciousness. These developments include the contributions made by the depth psychologies of Freud and Jung, the discovery of what have been called altered states of consciousness experienced and reported by many people (especially those who have used hallucinogenic drugs or have practised meditation), the influence of Eastern thought on a growing number of Western psychologists, etc. A leading figure among such psychologists, strongly influenced by Eastern thought, is Robert Ornstein who has resuscitated the early definition of psychology as the science of consciousness.[6]

When the early psychologists defined psychology as a science of consciousness, their view of consciousness was limited by the chief method which was then employed in psychology, namely, introspection. Consciousness was therefore conceived almost exclusively in terms of what was observable through mental introspection, which excluded all that lay outside mental awareness.

Recent years have witnessed not only the revival of interest in the study of consciousness but also in the deepening of the concept of consciousness. Ken Wilber, a noted present-day psychologist and a leading writer on the psychology of consciousness, has formulated such a deeper view of consciousness in his model of the "spectrum of consciousness". This model views the human being as a multi-levelled expression of a single consciousness, each level having its own characteristic sense of identity, ranging from the all-embracing infinite identity of cosmic consciousness to the exclusive, narrow identity of ego-consciousness. The innermost consciousness of the human being, states Wilber, "is identical to the absolute and ultimate reality of the universe" which is "spaceless

Self-Awareness

and therefore infinite, timeless and therefore eternal, outside of which nothing exists".[7] Compare this concept of consciousness with the erstwhile and still widely current view which, as Sri Aurobindo puts it, "sees consciousness only as a phenomenon that emerges out of inconscient Matter and consists of certain reactions of the system to outward things".[8] Wilber's concept echoes the yogic view of consciousness as "the Reality which is the very essence of existence"[9] about which Sri Aurobindo states:

> Consciousness is a fundamental thing, the fundamental thing in existence — it is the energy, the motion, the movement of consciousness that creates the universe and all that is in it — not only the macrocosm but the microcosm is nothing but consciousness arranging itself. For instance, when consciousness in its movement or rather a certain stress of movement forgets itself in the action it becomes an apparently "unconscious" energy; when it forgets itself in the form it becomes the electron, the atom, the material object. In reality it is still consciousness that works in the energy and determines the form and the evolution of form. When it wants to liberate itself, slowly, evolutionarily, out of Matter, but still in the form, it emerges as life, as animal, as man and it can go on evolving itself still farther out of its involution and become something more than mere man.[10]

What has been stated above regarding the yogic view of the nature of consciousness is meant to lead up to the yogic view of the nature of awareness. For, according to the psychology of yoga, awareness is an inherent element of consciousness. As Sri Aurobindo states: "Consciousness is made up of two elements, awareness of self and things and forces, and conscious-power."[11] Since, from the viewpoint of yoga, consciousness is the Reality, the very essence of existence and being, and since awareness is an element inherent in consciousness, to attain the fullness of existence and being is to be fully aware of one's being. This axiomatic truth is stated by Sri Aurobindo as follows:

> To be and to be fully is Nature's aim in us; but to be fully is to

be wholly conscious of one's being: unconsciousness, half consciousness or deficient consciousness is a state of being not in possession of itself; it is existence, but not fullness of being. To be aware wholly and integrally of oneself and of all the truth of one's being is the necessary condition of true possession of existence. This self-awareness is what is meant by spiritual knowledge....[12]

As pointed out previously, the enhancement of awareness of oneself is a striking parallel between several systems of modern psychology and psychotherapy on the one hand and yoga on the other. However, from what has just been quoted from Sri Aurobindo, it should be evident that the self-awareness spoken of and aimed at in yoga has a much more profound connotation, it being regarded as spiritual knowledge or knowledge of the essential truth of existence. For, from the viewpoint of yoga, Self and Existence are identical. In Sri Aurobindo's words:

Our supreme Self and the supreme Existence which has become the universe are one spirit, one self and one existence. The individual is in nature one expression of the universal Being, in spirit an emanation of the Transcendence. For if he finds his self, he finds too that his own true self is not this natural personality, this created individuality, but is a universal being in its relations with others and with Nature and in its upward term a portion or the living front of a supreme transcendental Spirit.[13]

The inextricable relationship that exists between what, from the viewpoint of modern psychology, appear to be disparate concepts, namely, consciousness, awareness and self, is expressed by Sri Aurobindo thus:

...the essence of consciousness is the power to be aware of itself and its objects.... Its true nature is to be wholly aware of its objects, and of these objects the first is self, the being which is evolving its consciousness here, and the rest is what we see as not-self,— but if existence is indivisible, that too must in reality be self: the destiny of evolving consciousness must be, then, to become perfect in its awareness, entirely aware of self and all-aware.[14]

One fundamental difference between the awareness aimed at in yoga and the insight fostered by analytical and other psychotherapeutic methods consists in the effective power for change which the awareness brings. It is a well-recognised fact in psychotherapy in general and in psychoanalysis in particular that most often mere insight in itself does not have an adequate impact for bringing about the needed changes in an individual's attitudes and behaviour. As it is said in psychoanalysis, in order to carry an effective power for bringing about a change, insight must be more than a mere intellectual perception; it must be an emotionally charged "corrective experience". And even after one has been led through psychoanalysis to such a genuine experience of one's unconscious psychodynamics, a more or less long process of "working through" is needed in order to translate the insight into behaviour. From the viewpoint of yoga, the explanation for the ineffectiveness of intellectual insight is to be found in what has been stated by Sri Aurobindo in a previous quotation regarding the fact that consciousness is made up of two elements — awareness and conscious-power or will-force. Each level of consciousness has its own characteristic type of awareness and degree of will-force. Intellectual awareness, which belongs to mental consciousness, is relatively ineffective because of the relative impotence of the will-force — the mental will-power — associated with it. As Sri Aurobindo observes:

> Those who live in the mind and the vital are not so well able to do this [call in the Force to make the change]; they are obliged to use mostly their personal effort and as the awareness and will and force of the mind and vital are divided and imperfect, the work done is imperfect and not definitive. It is only in the supermind* that Awareness, Will, Force are always one movement and automatically effective.[15]

* Sri Aurobindo uses the term "Supermind" to designate the principle supe-

In Yoga, on the other hand, the aim is to attain a progressively more evolved state of being than that of mental consciousness, thereby attaining a progressively greater force of one's being. To attain fullness of being, therefore, is not only, as previously stated by Sri Aurobindo, to be fully aware of one's being, but also to possess its full force. So Sri Aurobindo further states:

> But also, since consciousness carries in itself the force of existence, to be fully is to have the intrinsic and integral force of one's being; it is to come into possession of all one's force of self and of all its use. To be merely, without possessing the force of one's being or with a half-force or deficient force of it, is a mutilated or diminished existence; it is to exist, but it is not fullness of being.[16]

There is yet another essential characteristic of the self-awareness sought in yoga which distinguishes it from the kind of awareness of oneself obtained through psychotherapy. The ultimate aim of all psychotherapy is to lead to psychological well-being. However, in most cases, the awareness gained through psychotherapy does not in itself bring about the state of total well-being. In yoga, on the other hand, the essence of Being is conceived of as Sachchidananda, a trinity of Existence (*sat*), Consciousness (*cit*) and Delight or Bliss (*ānanda*). Therefore, to attain fullness of being and existence is to attain not only the full awareness and the full force of one's being, but also its full delight, which is the highest consummation of psychological well-being. To quote Sri Aurobindo:

> Lastly, to be fully is to have the full delight of being. Being without delight of being, without an entire delight of itself and all things is something neutral or diminished; it is existence, but it is not fullness of being.... All undelight, all pain and suffering are a sign of imperfection, of incompleteness; they arise

---

rior to Mind; Supermind is the Truth-Consciousness which "exists, acts and proceeds in the fundamental truth and unity of things and not like the mind in their appearances and phenomenal divisions." (*The Life Divine*, SABCL, Vol. 18, p. 143)

Self-Awareness

from a division of being, an incompleteness of consciousness of being, an incompleteness of the force of being. To become complete in being, in consciousness of being, in force of being, in delight of being and to live in this integrated completeness is the divine living.[17]

REFERENCES

1. Fritjof Capra, *The Tao of Physics*. Boston & London: New Science Library, Shambhala, 1983.
2. Albert Ellis, "Rational-Emotive Therapy" in Virginia Binder, Arnold Binder & Bernard Rimland (Eds.) *Modern Therapies*. New Jersey: Prentice-Hall, Inc., 1976, pp. 22-23.
3. Sri Aurobindo, *Letters on Yoga*, Sri Aurobindo Birth Centenary Library (hereafter SABCL) (Pondicherry: Sri Aurobindo Ashram, 1970-75), Vol. 22, p. 233.
4. The Mother, *Collected Works of the Mother* (Pondicherry: Sri Aurobindo Ashram, 1978), Vol. 12, p. 3.
5. Sri Aurobindo, *Letters on Yoga*, SABCL, Vol. 24, p. 1394.
6. Robert Ornstein, *The Psychology of Consciousness*. San Francisco: W. H. Freeman, 1972.
7. Ken Wilber, "*Psychologia Perennis*: The Spectrum of Consciousness" in John Welwood (Ed.), *The Meeting of the Ways*. New York: Schocken Books, 1979, pp. 8-9.
8. Sri Aurobindo, *Letters on Yoga*, SABCL, Vol. 22, p. 238.
9. Ibid.
10. Ibid., pp. 236-37.
11. Ibid., p. 238.
12. Sri Aurobindo, *The Life Divine*, SABCL, Vol. 19, pp. 1023-24.
13. Sri Aurobindo, *The Synthesis of Yoga*, SABCL, Vol. 20, p. 282.
14. Sri Aurobindo, *The Life Divine*, SABCL, Vol. 19, p. 1017.
15. Sri Aurobindo, *Letters on Yoga*, SABCL, Vol. 22, p. 238.
16. Sri Aurobindo, *The Life Divine*, SABCL, Vol. 19, p. 1024.
17. Ibid., pp. 1024-25.

4 THE NATURE OF IDENTIFICATION

Identification is regarded by many psychologists as an important concept for understanding both the early development of personality and its later growth. However, from the viewpoint of yoga psychology, identification is a much more pervasive and deeper phenomenon, of which only some limited and superficial aspects are recognised in modern psychology. This essay aims at explicating the deeper nature of identification as viewed in Integral Yoga psychology.

As a psychological concept, identification has several different though related meanings and implications. These various meanings and implications of the term may be understood by considering the different forms of identification.

Forms of Ordinary Identification

Common forms of identification which are generally recognized fall into four categories:

1. *Identification with persons:* Two main forms of identification in relation to persons may be distinguished:

(a) Identification with an idealized person, or someone who is strongly admired, such as a parent, a teacher, a hero, a star, and the like. The general psychological definition of identification as a process by which one incorporates in oneself aspects of another's personality applies to this form of identification. It implies an unconscious tendency to *become like* the other person who constitutes, in the language of psychology, an aspect of one's ego-ideal. Identification in this sense is in a way similar to emulation, but whereas the former is mostly an unconscious process, the latter involves conscious effort.

It is in a somewhat similar sense that Freud — perhaps the first theorist in the West to write about identification — used the concept in explaining the origin of his construct of the super-ego or conscience. According to him, the super-ego is the result of identification with the parent and the consequent introjection of parental values.

(b) Identification with relatives, friends and other similar relationships based on love, affection or liking. Such identification, depending on its degree or extent, results in an unconscious tendency to *think, feel and act in sympathy* with the person one is identified with, as if the other person were an extension of oneself. Good and bad fortunes of the other person are felt, in varying degrees, as if they were one's own good and bad fortunes.

Identification with a group with which one is affiliated, such as a club, society, political party, nation, etc. also falls under this category.

2. *Identification with descriptive characteristics of oneself:*

A person is identified in society by various descriptive particulars, such as the person's name, caste, religion, nationality, race, occupation, etc. Identification with such descriptive labels of oneself implies that the descriptive characteristic is an *integral part of one's self-concept*; one's idea of oneself is inextricably associated with the description. The feeling of narcissism or love of oneself is therefore unconsciously extended to the name, caste, religion, etc. with which one is identified. Feelings of pride or shame regarding any of one's descriptive characteristics equally betray an identification.

3. *Identification with parts or aspects of oneself:*

Identification with one's body, feelings and impulses, or the mind and its thoughts comes under this category. Such identifications imply that the part one identifies with is regarded *the same as oneself.* Consequently, the states, activities and reactions of that part are felt as one's own states, activities and reactions. For instance, if the body is ill, the person feels and says, "I am ill"; when a thought occurs to the mind, the person says, "I think", etc. This form of identification is spoken of mostly in Indian psychology, though it is also recognized by some thinkers in the West, such as Roberto Assagioli, founder of the psychotherapeutic system called Psychosynthesis.

Carl Jung, the Swiss psychiatrist, has written about identification with a personality trait, such as extroversion or introversion, masculinity or femininity, etc. Such identification with an aspect of oneself may be subsumed under this category. It implies that the trait one identifies with is regarded as an *essential characteristic of oneself*; consequently, one unconsciously acts in terms of that trait.

4. *Identification with one's possessions:*

Identification with possessions is indicated by the very sense of ownership in relation to them. The sense of ownership implies that the possession is regarded as a *psychological appendage of oneself*. Consequently, one is affected by what affects the possessions. Thus praise or criticism of a possession is felt as praise or criticism of oneself; damage to a possession causes hurt as if the damage were to oneself.

Characteristics of Ordinary Identification

The chief psychological characteristics of the common forms of identification just described are as follows:

(a) The central characteristic of identification is implied in the etymological root of the term: *idem*, which means 'the same'. Identification therefore implies that the thing or person or trait or part one identifies with is considered, in varying degrees, to be *the same as oneself*. In terms of Indian psychology, the separate self or the ego is the basis of identification; the ego is extended in varying degrees to embrace the object of one's identification which in some measure is regarded to be the same as oneself.

(b) Since what one identifies with is an extension of one's ego, the ego's inherent love of itself is extended to the thing or person or trait or part one identifies with. Thus the common forms of identification are characterized by *attachment* to the object of identification.

(c) Identification is an *unconscious process* and leads to *involuntary emotional reactions* associated with the object of one's identification. It is said to be an unconscious process because one can become aware of it only *after* it has been formed. The associated emotional reactions are involuntary in the sense that one cannot help experiencing the *feelings* involved, even if one can prevent one's *thinking* and *actions* from being influenced by the identification. For instance, when a close friend has a conflict with a third person, one cannot help feeling a predilection in favour of the friend, in spite of the fact that, rationally, one may regard the third person as being in the right and may actually take a stand in favour of the third person.

In the light of what has been stated above regarding the characteristics of the common forms of identification, it is not surprising that in psychotherapy emphasis has come to be placed almost exclusively on the negative aspects of identification. When psychotherapists refer to identification, it is almost always to point out the need for dis-identification in order to free oneself from the influence of unconscious identifications which bind and limit the individual.

From the viewpoint of the deeper psychology of Integral Yoga, however, there are two types of identification — one which leads to ignorance and bondage, and one that leads to knowledge and freedom.

Two Types of Identification

The two kinds of identification are alluded to in the following passage:

> Consciousness is the faculty of becoming aware of anything whatsoever through identification with it. But the divine consciousness is not only aware but knows and effects. For mere awareness is not knowledge.... Only when the consciousness participates in the divine consciousness does it get full knowledge by identification with the object. Ordinarily, identification leads to ignorance rather than to knowledge, for the consciousness is lost in what it becomes and is unable to envisage proper causes, concomitants and consequences. Thus you identify yourself with a movement of anger and your whole being becomes one angry vibration, blind and precipitate, oblivious of everything else. It is only when you stand back, remain detached in the midst of the passionate turmoil that you

are able to see the process with a knowing eye. So knowledge in the ordinary state of being is to be obtained rather by stepping back from a phenomenon, to watch it without becoming identified with it. But the divine consciousness identifies itself with its object and knows it thoroughly, because it always becomes one with the essential truth or law inherent in each fact.[1]

The passage contains two profound implications regarding the nature of identification:

(a) It is through some degree of identification that one becomes aware of anything. In other words, to become aware of a thing is, in some measure, to identify with it, that is, become one with it in one's consciousness. Thus there is some degree of identification with everything that we come in contact with and become aware of. The Mother states this fact more explicitly in speaking about the dispersion of consciousness. She says:

> One is always identified more or less with all that one does and all the things with which one is in contact. The ordinary state of people is to be in everything that they do, all that they see, all whom they frequently meet.[2]

The subtle truth that the very awareness of a thing implies some degree of identification with it is more easily comprehensible in relation to feelings and emotions. From a psychological viewpoint, to be able to understand truly another person's feelings, one must empathize or *feel with* the other person. In other words, to become aware of another person's feelings, one must identify or become one with the other person's feelings. Thus at bottom, identification is a reflection of what in yoga has been called knowledge by identity — the highest form of knowledge which consists in becoming one with the object to be known. Sri Aurobindo has stated it thus:

> In reality, all experience is in its secret nature knowledge by identity; but its true character is hidden from us because we have separated ourselves from the rest of the world by exclusion, by the distinction of our self as subject and everything

else as object, and we are compelled to develop processes and organs by which we may again enter into communion with all that we have excluded. We have to replace direct knowledge through conscious identity by an individual knowledge which appears to be caused by physical contact and mental sympathy.[3]

From what has been stated above, it follows that hidden behind all the forms of identification normal to human beings there is the secret knowledge by identity possessed by the innermost self. The commonly recognized forms of identification mentioned earlier are only the external and more obvious forms of a subtle and all-pervasive process which, for the most part, is veiled to our surface awareness. Identification in its essential sense is thus a much deeper and wider process than what it is believed to be in modern psychology.

(b) The second implication pertains to the double nature of identification and the distinction that exists between the two types of identification. The ordinary type of identification leads to ignorance, "for the consciousness is lost in what it becomes"; to the extent one identifies with a thing, one becomes "oblivious of everything else". The other type of identification leads to knowledge because consciousness "becomes one with the essential truth or law inherent in each fact". The Mother alludes to this latter type of identification when she says: "I know the character of a man through self-identification.... *all* knowledge is knowledge by identification. That is, one must become that which one wants to know."[4]

The key to the paradox that identification results in ignorance as well as knowledge lies in understanding the relationship between the two types of identification mentioned above. This relationship is very similar to the relationship between desire and love, which has been well brought out in the following remarks of the Mother:

> I believe, right at its origin it [desire] is an obscure need for growth, as in the lowest forms of life love is changed into the need to swallow, absorb, become joined with another thing.

> This is the most primitive form of love in the lowest forms of life, it is to take and absorb. Well, the need to take is desire. So perhaps if we went far back enough into the last depths of the inconscience, we could say that the origin of desire is love. It is love in its obscurest and most unconscious form. It is a need to become joined with something....[5]

The identification which leads to ignorance may in similar terms be described as identification in its obscurest, most unconscious and most primitive form. The Mother alludes to its primitive nature in speaking about identification with one's possessions. She says:

> ...people — the ones I call altogether primitive — are attached to things: when they have something, they do not want to let it go! It seems so childish to me!... When they have to part with something, it hurts! Because they identify themselves with the things they have....[6]

As stated earlier, attachment is one of the chief characteristics of the common forms of identification. On the other hand, the identification that leads to knowledge is characterized by a complete absence of attachment. As the Mother states:

> ...a perfect indifference and neutrality is the indispensable condition for a knowledge by integral identity. If there be a single detail, however small, which escapes the neutrality, that detail escapes also the identification. Therefore, the absence of all personal reaction,... is a primary necessity for a total knowledge.
>
> One can thus say, paradoxically, that we can know a thing only when we are not interested in it, or rather, more exactly, when we are not personally concerned with it.[7]

The Mother alludes to the two types of identification in another context where she speaks about the need to accumulate things. She says:

They [human beings] sense their limitation and think that in order to grow, increase and even survive, they need to take things from outside, for they live in the consciousness of their personal limitation... Naturally, this is a mistake. And the truth is that if instead of being shut up in the narrow limits of their little person, they could so widen their consciousness as to be able not only to identify themselves with others in their narrow limits, but to come out of these limits, pass beyond, spread out everywhere, unite with the one Consciousness and become all things, then, at that moment the narrow limits will vanish, but not before. And as long as one senses the narrow limits, one wants to take, for one fears to lose.... One tries to take, accumulate, accumulate, accumulate, but that is impossible, one can't accumulate. One must identify oneself.... The more one spreads out, the more one has. The more one gets identified, the more one becomes. And then, instead of taking, one gives. And the more one gives, the more one grows.

But for this one must be able to come out of the limits of one's little ego. One must be identified with the Force, identified with the Vibration instead of being identified with one's ego.[8]

The fundamental difference between the two types of identification is implied in the above-quoted passage. One type of identification involves being "identified with one's ego"; in the other type of identification one "must be able to come out of the limits of one's little ego". The former type is illustrated by the common forms of identification, the central characteristic of which, as stated earlier, is that they are related to the ego. Identifications which partake of the nature of the latter type, too, occur in ordinary life, although they take place unconsciously and are not usually recognized as phenomena of identification. The Mother gives several everyday examples of identification in which one forgets the ego:

For instance, when you are reading a book that interests you very much, a wonderful novel full of exciting adventures, when you are completely absorbed in the story,... this is a phenomenon of self-identification. And if you do it with a certain perfection, you succeed in understanding ahead what is going to happen. There is a moment when, being fully absorbed in the story, you come to know (without trying to look for it) towards what end the author is leading you.... For you have identified yourself with the creative thought of the author. You do it more or less perfectly, without knowing that you are doing it....

These are phenomena of self-identification. Only, they are involuntary. And this is also one of the methods used today to cure nervous diseases. When someone cannot sleep, cannot be restful because he is too excited and nervous and his nerves are ill and weakened by excessive agitation, he is told to sit in front of an aquarium... and look at the fish. So he looks at the fish, moving around, coming and going, swimming, gliding, turning, meeting, crossing, chasing one another indefinitely.... After a while he lives the life of fishes: he comes and goes, swims, glides, plays. And at the end of the hour his nerves are in a perfect state and he is completely restful![9]

Conscious Identification

As stated previously, one of the characteristics of the common forms of identification involving the ego is that it is an unconscious process. The examples just cited show that the salutary type of identification in which one forgets the ego can, too, take place unconsciously. However, whereas the former type of identification is necessarily unconscious, the latter can be learnt consciously. This is stated by the Mother in commenting on Sri Aurobindo's statement: "Knowledge can only come by conscious identity, for that is the only true knowledge — existence aware of itself."[10] The Mother comments as follows:

> There is always some kind of *unconscious identification* with the surrounding people and things; but by will and practice one can learn to concentrate on somebody or something and to get consciously identified with this person or this thing, and

through this identification you know the nature of the person or the thing.[11]

The Mother has spoken about several methods for learning how to identify oneself consciously with a thing or person. Two particular methods which she has recommended on several occasions are described here.

One method consists in concentrating on an object, or a drawing of a design, or simply a point:

> ...it is very convenient to take a point: one looks steadily at the point, and so steadily that at a certain moment one becomes the point. One is no longer somebody looking at the point; one is the point. And then, if you continue with sufficient strength and quietness, without anything disturbing you, you may suddenly find yourself before a door which opens and you pass to the other side. And then you have the revelation.[12]

Another method consists in trying to enter the mind of another person with whom one disagrees about something. The Mother describes the method thus:

> ...instead of doing that [arguing],... if you tell yourself: "Wait a little, I am going to try and see why he said that to me".... And you concentrate: "Why, why, why?"... you concentrate more and more on what he is saying, and with the feeling that gradually, through his words, you are entering his mind. When you enter his head, suddenly you enter into his way of thinking....
> ...if you make that little movement, and instead of looking at him as an object quite alien to you, you try to enter within, you enter within, into that little head that's before you, and then, suddenly, you find yourself on the other side, you look at yourself and understand quite well what he is saying — everything is clear, the why, the how, the reason, the feeling which is behind the whole thing....[13]

The Mother, however, points out that knowledge about a thing or a person through identification with that thing or person is not the same as knowledge of the thing or of the person through identifying with the Supreme Reality. She says:

> ...by unity with the Supreme you share the Supreme Nature and get the full knowledge whenever you turn to observe any object and identify yourself with it... which is certainly more than what is called in yogic parlance knowledge by identity. For, the kind of identification taught by many disciplines extends your limits of perception without piercing to the innermost heart of an object: it sees from within it, as it were, but only its phenomenal aspect. For example, if you identify yourself with a tree, you become aware in the way in which a tree is aware of itself, yet you do not come to know everything about a tree.[14]

The Mother was once asked: Can one attain the Divine by learning how to identify consciously? This is how she replied:

> ...the only way of knowing the Divine is by identifying oneself with Him.... Hence, once you are master of this method of identification, you can identify yourself.... But so long as you do not know how to identify yourself, a hundred and one things will always come across your path, pulling you here, pulling you there, scattering you, and you will not be able to identify yourself with Him. But if you have learnt how to identify yourself, then you have only to orientate the identification, place it where you want it, and then hold on there until you get a result. It will come very fast if you are master of your power of identification.[15]

REFERENCES

1. The Mother, *Collected Works of the Mother* (Pondicherry: Sri Aurobindo Ashram, 1972-1987), Vol. 3, p. 167.
2. The Mother, *Collected Works of the Mother*, Vol. 7, p. 256.
3. Sri Aurobindo, *The Life Divine*, Sri Aurobindo Birth Centenary Library (hereafter SABCL) (Pondicherry: Sri Aurobindo Ashram, 1970-75), Vol. 18, p. 62.

4. The Mother, *Collected Works of the Mother*, Vol. 5, p. 219.
5. The Mother, *Collected Works of the Mother*, Vol. 7, pp. 37-38.
6. The Mother, *Collected Works of the Mother*, Vol. 10, p. 174.
7. The Mother, *Collected Works of the Mother*, Vol. 15, p. 299.
8. The Mother, *Collected Works of the Mother*, Vol. 5, pp. 233-34.
9. Ibid., pp. 223-24.
10. Sri Aurobindo, *The Life Divine*, SABCL, Vol. 18, p. 213.
11. The Mother, *Collected Works of the Mother*, Vol. 14, pp. 51-52.
12. The Mother, *Collected Works of the Mother*, Vol. 5, p. 400.
13. Ibid., pp. 221-22.
14. The Mother, *Collected Works of the Mother*, Vol. 3, pp. 167-68.
15. The Mother, *Collected Works of the Mother*, Vol. 5, p. 225.

PART TWO

MENTAL HEALTH AND YOGA

There is a psychological health just as there is a physical health.

THE MOTHER

It is only by a change — not a mere readjustment — of man's present nature that it can be developed, and such a change is not possible except by yoga.

SRI AUROBINDO

5 MENTAL HEALTH AND SRI AUROBINDO'S INTEGRAL YOGA

The term "mental health", so widely used today, especially in the West, seems to be conspicuous by its absence in almost all spiritual disciplines. The focus of spiritual disciplines has been on overcoming the illusion of the separate self, the realization of the true Self and the attainment of Enlightenment rather than on the achievement of mental health. During the past few decades, numerous concepts and values related to spirituality, hitherto more or less unknown or tabooed in science and the academe, have entered the thought and language of psychology and psychiatry with increasing ease and frequency. Examples of such concepts and values are: altered states of consciousness, consciousness raising, higher consciousness, the transpersonal, the Higher Self, psychosynthesis, self-actualization; living in the here and now, meditation, centredness, etc. The spiritual nuance in the current thinking about mental health was brought home strikingly to the present writer by the editorial of an issue of the Oregon Mental Health Association Newsletter where mental health was defined as peace of mind!

The fact that concepts of the spiritual life are gaining currency in the field of mental health points to some relationship that must exist between spirituality and mental health. The purpose of this essay is to explicate this relationship in the light of Sri Aurobindo's Integral Yoga. In order to do this, we will draw upon those teachings of Sri Aurobindo and the Mother which relate to some of the basic parameters of mental health, such as the meaning of mental health, aetiological factors which undermine mental health, and ways of achieving mental health. In the course of such an exposition of the mental health teachings implicit in Integral Yoga, we will note some of the similarities and differences between the commonly accepted concepts of mental health and those of Integral Yoga.

Meaning of Mental Health

What is believed to constitute mental health is intimately related to what is believed to be the nature of the human being. A theory of psychopathology, dealing with the origin and nature of psychological disturbances, always rests, implicitly or explicitly, on a certain personality theory pertaining to the psychological structure, development and functioning of the human being.

According to Integral Yoga, a human being is made up of many different parts which function on different levels of consciousness and express different types of consciousness. Very broadly speaking, a human being is regarded as a soul or psyche, using mind, life and body for its self-discovery and manifestation. Each part of the being — psychic, mental, vital, physical — has its own separate and distinct consciousness, though interconnected and interacting with the rest. Because of the interactions among the parts of the being, there exist subdivisions in each part of the being. Thus, with regard to mind, there is a mind proper (the thinking mind), a physical mind (the part of the mind which is influenced by the consciousness of the physical), a vital mind (the part of the mind influenced by the vital), and a psychic mind (the part of the mind acted upon by the psychic). The same subdivisions exist within the physical and vital planes of the being. Each subdivision has its own typical consciousness and modes of activity. This makes a human being a highly complex creature who is constantly pushed and pulled by many, often conflicting, forces. The more developed an individual is, the greater the complexity of the being. Speaking of this, Nolini Kanta Gupta makes the following remarks based on a talk of the Mother:

> Man does not live on a single plane but on many planes at the same time. There is a scale of gradation in human consciousness: the higher one rises in the scale the greater the number of elements or personalities that one possesses. Whether one lives mostly or mainly on the physical or vital or mental plane or on any particular section of these planes or on planes above and beyond, there will be accordingly differences in the constitu-

tion or psycho-physical make-up of the individual personality. The higher one stands the richer the personality, because it lives not only on its own normal level, but also on all that are below and which it has transcended. The complete or integral man, some occultists say, possesses 365 personalities; indeed it may be much more.[1]

The view of human nature as a complexity of different parts or systems is expressed in several modern personality theories. Among these theories, the system of psychosynthesis, formulated by Assagioli, which speaks of an individual as made up of various aspects of the self and numerous subpersonalities, provides perhaps the greatest elaboration of human nature as a composite of different parts. However, compared to the description of the parts of the being found in Integral Yoga — only the broadest outlines of which have been presented above — the psychosynthesis view of human personality would appear much less profound and quite incomplete.

Given such a view of our nature, we are faced with two basic problems. One is the great difficulty in understanding ourselves. A good deal of the time we do not know why we feel or act the way we do, because we do not know which part of our being is responsible for our feeling or our act. Not knowing the springs of our thoughts, feelings and actions, we are naturally incapable of intelligently controlling or directing them.

The second problem arising out of the complex make-up of our nature is the inevitable conflict among the different parts of the being. It is therefore not surprising that most psychological disturbances are seen to involve some forms of inner conflict.

In the light of what we have just said, mental health depends, first and foremost, on the extent to which one is conscious of the different parts of one's being so as to be able to exercise self-mastery and self-direction, rather than be pulled hither and thither by strings whose origins one is not aware of. Secondly, mental health depends on the measure of unification that one can bring about among the different parts of one's being so as to replace conflict and strife by harmony and peace.

To be conscious of the different parts of one's being and to be able to unify them, one needs to discover the inmost centre of oneself, the psychic being. According to Integral Yoga, what prevents such a discovery is an identification with one's outer being of body, life and mind. All the psychological disturbances which sap mental health are ultimately attributable to the limitations, imperfections and ignorance inherent in the very nature of these instruments of our being. Some of the chief disturbances related to the mental, vital and physical planes of our being are pointed out below.*

Disturbances of the Mental

As noted above, each part of our being interacts with and is influenced by other parts, making for subdivisions in each part. The part of the mind which is influenced by physical consciousness has been called the physical mind. The mechanical and senseless mental repetitions which we all experience in varying degrees, and which become pronounced to a pathological degree in some types of obsessive thinking, are a feature of an aspect of the physical mind which is called the mechanical mind. The Mother gives some examples of the activity of the mechanical mind:

> For example, you see, if it fancies counting: "One, two, three, four", then it will go on: "One, two, three, four; one, two, three, four." And you may think of all kinds of things, but it goes on: "One, two, three, four", like that... Or it catches hold of three words, four words and repeats them and goes on repeating them; and unless one turns away with a certain violence and punches it soundly telling it, "Keep quiet!", it continues in this way, indefinitely.[2]

Readers who are familiar with the technique of "thought stopping" employed in behaviour therapy will note the striking similarity

---

* These disturbances are presented in greater detail in a subsequent essay, "Psychological Disturbances: A Model Based on Sri Aurobindo's Yoga".

between this technique and the method recommended by the Mother for stopping obsessive thoughts.

Another disturbance caused by the physical mind, also recognized in the field of mental health, is related to its tendency towards doubt, leading to perpetual uncertainty. This is due to the obscurity of the physical consciousness as it affects the mind. All of us experience this doubt and uncertainty of the physical mind in varying degrees, though it strikes us only when it manifests to an abnormal degree as in some of the compulsions of the obsessive-compulsive neurosis, e.g. the compulsion to check and re-check if a door has been locked or whether the gas has been turned off.

But perhaps the greatest disturbance of the physical mind comes from its susceptibility to the things and circumstances of the physical plane which provoke it to ceaseless and incoherent activity. This subjection to the physical world turns the mind into a factory of thoughts and a public square where thoughts constantly come and go, without any order, coherence or organization. Because of our identification with the physical mind, we believe that it is *we* who create the thoughts, whereas in fact the thoughts are produced in us by external factors. Our efforts at controlling our thoughts are futile precisely because our thoughts originate outside our being.

It is relatively recently that the restless activity of the physical mind has begun to draw the attention of mental health practitioners. However, if mental health is regarded as consisting of peace of mind, the restlessness of the physical mind would be seen as one of the most fundamental problems of mental health.

Another subdivision of the mind noted above is the vital mind. The vast majority of mankind have evolved beyond the predominantly vital consciousness that governs animal behaviour, but have not yet actualized the truly mental nature, the rational mind. The predominant level of consciousness in most human beings, therefore, is that of the vital mind. One manifestation of the vital mind which is particularly relevant to mental health is to be seen in what have been called defense mechanisms which characterize all neurotic and psychotic disturbances. A principal defense mechanism is that of rationalization by which the mind conspires with the vital and gives rational explanations for actions which are in fact based on impulses and desires of the vital. Sri Aurobindo states:

> The vital started in its evolution with obedience to impulse and no reason.... It does not like the voice of knowledge and wisdom — but curiously enough by the necessity which has grown up in man of justifying action by reason, the *vital mind* has developed a strategy of its own which is to get the reason to find out reasons for justifying its own feelings and impulses.[3]

The fundamental cause of all psychological disturbances, however, lies in the very nature of mind with the objectivising or reflective nature of its consciousness. As the Mother observes:

> It is obvious that what especially characterises man is this mental capacity of watching himself live. The animal lives spontaneously, automatically, and if it watches itself live, it must be to a very minute and insignificant degree, and that is why it is peaceful and does not worry. Even if an animal is suffering because of an accident or an illness, this suffering is reduced to a minimum by the fact that it does not observe it, does not project it in its consciousness and into the future, does not imagine things about its illness or its accident.
>
> With man there has begun this perpetual worrying about what is going to happen, and this worry is the principal, if not the sole cause of his torment. With this objectivising consciousness there has begun anxiety, painful imaginations, worry, torment, anticipation of future catastrophes, with the result that most men — and not the least conscious, the most conscious — live in perpetual torment. Man is too conscious to be indifferent, he is not conscious enough to know what will happen....
>
> How can a problem be solved when one doesn't have the necessary knowledge? And the unfortunate thing is that man believes that he has to resolve all the problems of his life, and he does not have the knowledge needed to do it. That is the source, the origin of all his troubles — that perpetual question, "What should I do?" which is followed by another one still more acute, "What is going to happen?" and at the same time, more or less, the inability to answer.[4]

The metapsychological basis of what the existential psychotherapists have called *Angst* (anxiety) is contained in the above-quoted passage.

Disturbances of the Vital

The vital corresponds somewhat to what in Western psychology has been called the libido — not in the narrow, sexual connotation given to the term by Freud, but in the broad sense in which Jung used it to connote the source of all energies. From the viewpoint of Integral Yoga, most human beings in their evolutionary growth have not yet fully emerged into the mental principle, and are therefore still chiefly governed by the vital. This may be seen from the fact that one of the chief characteristics of the vital, namely, the pursuit of pleasure (related to the "pleasure principle", as Freud called it), with its concomitant avoidance of pain, constitutes a prime motivator of human behaviour. As the Mother remarks: "...one of the two principal occupations of man is to try to forget what is painful to him, and the other is to try to seek amusement in order to escape boredom."[5]

Most of the psychological disturbances that have been identified and labelled in the field of mental health are ultimately attributable to the principle of desire inherent in the vital. For the two chief factors which are found to underlie all functional psychiatric disorders, namely, anxiety and depression, are related to the vital. A third destroyer of mental health — anger — is also a chief manifestation of the vital. Though not yet universally recognized as detrimental to mental health, anger, according to one medical authority, is at the basis of half of all psychosomatic illnesses. The following observations made by the Mother point to the psychodynamics of anger and depression as viewed in Integral Yoga:

> ...one is almost constantly in an ordinary vital state where the least unpleasant thing very spontaneously and easily brings you depression — depression if you are a weak person, revolt if you are a strong one. Every desire which is not satisfied, every impulse which meets an obstacle, every unpleasant contact with

outside things, very easily and very spontaneously creates depression or revolt...⁶

The dynamics of anger and depression as stated above can be better understood when these two feeling-states are seen as the psychological correlates of the well-known "fight or flight" response spoken of in psychology. An important implication of this correlation is that anger, which is associated with the sympathetic reaction of the fighting response, is necessarily a stress producing reaction, even though anger is often not recognised as detrimental by mental health professionals.

One specific form of vital disturbance which has gained attention in the field of behavioural medicine during the recent past is what has been called "time urgency". This trait of "hurry sickness" has been identified as one of the chief characteristics of Type A behaviour* which, according to the well-known studies of Friedman and Rosenman, constitutes the major cause of America's number one killer — coronary artery and heart disease. This aspect of Type A behaviour and its consequence are well described by the Mother.

> We — I mean men — live harassed lives. It is a kind of half-awareness of the shortness of their lives; they do not think of it, but they feel it half-consciously. And so they are always wanting — quick, quick, quick — to rush from one thing to another, to do one thing quickly and move on to the next one, instead of letting each thing live in its own eternity. They are always wanting: forward, forward, forward.... You go hurtling through life... to go where?... You end with a crash!⁷

Disturbances of the Physical

Whereas the vital is governed by the principle of desire or Rajas, the physical consciousness is characterized by inertia or Tamas.

---

* A label given to a typical cluster of behavioural characteristics the central feature of which is a drive to achieve the maximum within the shortest possible time, leading to time urgency, aggressive competitiveness and other related behaviours.

An individual who lives chiefly in the physical consciousness needs strong and violent stimulation in order to overcome the deadweight of inertia and feel "alive". Describing such individuals the Mother says:

> ...they always need new excitements, dramas, murders, suicides, etc. to get the impression of something... For it is this need of excitement which shakes you up a little, makes you come out of yourself.[8]

What is experienced as a pleasant stimulation by the average person — in whom the vital, rajasic consciousness is predominant — is too dull and feeble to produce a reaction in the individual whose consciousness is predominantly tamasic. What is capable of producing a reaction in such a person is an extremely strong stimulation which the average person would experience as unpleasant or even painful. In the field of mental health this condition has been called masochism — a state in which what is generally experienced as painful is felt to be pleasurable. Thus the masochistic disorders spoken of in psychiatry seem to be related to the physical consciousness.

Because of the interaction between different parts of the being mentioned earlier, various disturbances of the physical manifest in the mind and the vital since the physical consciousness affects the mental and the vital. Some of the disturbances of the physical as they affect the mind have been noted above in referring to the physical mind.

Achieving Mental Health

The field of mental health abounds with numerous psychotherapeutic approaches for achieving mental health. All these approaches may be classified into three broad categories according as they focus on the body (including life energy), the feelings or the mind in attempting to bring about change in the direction of what is regarded as mental health. The body therapies range from the grossly physical approaches, such as chemotherapy and electroshock therapy, to psycho-physical methods such as Bioenergetics, Rolfing, Shiatsu, etc. Gestalt therapy is the leader among the therapies that focus on feelings. Rational-Emotive therapy, psychoanalysis and other analytical therapies work primarily with the mind. While the focus may be different, all the psychotherapeutic approaches have the common objective of making a person *feel* better, because as we have previously stated, almost all the psychological disturbances involve the vital or feeling-nature.

The focus in Integral Yoga is on the psyche, the inmost part of the being. The aim is to unify the being by organizing all the parts of the being around the psychic centre. The state in which this process of unification culminates is that of yoga or union with the Self, since the psyche is the individual representative of the supreme and universal Self. "When we have this realisation," says Sri Aurobindo, "when we dwell in it securely and permanently, all possibilities of grief and sin, fear, delusion, internal strife and pain are driven puissantly from our being."[9] Such a state, which is not only totally but also permanently free from all psychological disturbances, evidently far transcends the state of mental health as generally conceived.

It may be said that from the perspective of Integral Yoga psychology, psychotherapy is to the vital what medical science is to the body; each of these two fields aims at healing the maladies of a particular part of the being. However, the premise of Integral Yoga, as of all spiritual disciplines, is that true healing, as the etymology of the term implies, can come about only when the division and discord among the members of the being are replaced by wholeness and harmony. Therefore, the commonly practised mental health approaches, whose objective is to heal a specific part of the being, can at best bring about only a temporary adjustment and a partial alleviation of suffering, chiefly in the vital. The radical change that is called for in the physical, vital, and mental consciousness before the being is unified can be effected only by a spiritual discipline. As Sri Aurobindo puts it: "...it is only by a change — not a mere readjustment — of man's present nature that it can be developed, and such a change is not possible except by yoga."[10]

Summary and Conclusions

The increasing percolation of spiritual concepts and terms into the field of psychology and psychiatry points to a relationship between spirituality and mental health. The purpose of this essay has been to explicate this relationship in the light of the psychological thought implicit in Sri Aurobindo's Yoga. To this end, some of the basic teachings of Sri Aurobindo and the Mother as they relate to mental health have been explained with reference to the meaning of mental health, aetiological factors underlying psychological disturbances, and ways of achieving mental health. Some similarities and differences between Integral Yoga and current thought in the field of mental health have been pointed out.

Both modern personality theories and Integral Yoga allude to the great complexity of the human make-up. By and large, mental health approaches have sought to deal with the disturbances of what in Integral Yoga is called the vital. Therefore, in the light of Integral Yoga, mental health approaches are fraught with two basic limitations. In the first place, such approaches address themselves largely to the disturbances of only one part of the being, namely, the vital nature, not recognizing that the physical and the mental parts of consciousness also are sources of psychological disturbances. Secondly, mental health approaches do not recognize the fact that psychological disturbances are inherent in the very constitutional nature of physical, vital and mental consciousness. Therefore the attempt to obtain freedom from the disturbances of the physical, the vital, and the mental while one is still identified with these inherently afflicted parts of the being can at best lead to a temporary and superficial sense of well-being. It is only the discovery of the psychic being that can bring abiding peace and happiness.

REFERENCES

1. Nolini Kanta Gupta, *Yoga of Sri Aurobindo*, Part Six (Pondicherry: Sri Aurobindo Ashram, 1972), p. 238.
2. The Mother, *Collected Works of the Mother* (Pondicherry: Sri Aurobindo Ashram, 1972-1987), Vol. 6, p. 319.

3. Sri Aurobindo, *Letters on Yoga*, Sri Aurobindo Birth Centenary Library (hereafter SABCL) (Pondicherry: Sri Aurobindo Ashram, 1970-1975), Vol. 24, p. 1329.
4. The Mother, *Collected Works of the Mother* Vol. 9, pp. 303-4.
5. The Mother, *Collected Works of the Mother* Vol. 4, p. 205.
6. The Mother, *Collected Works of the Mother*, Vol. 8, p. 192.
7. The Mother, *Collected Works of the Mother*, Vol. 10, pp. 202-3.
8. The Mother, *Collected Works of the Mother*, Vol. 5, p. 415.
9. Sri Aurobindo, *The Yoga and Its Objects*, SABCL, Vol. 16, p. 417.
10. Ibid., pp. 412-13.

6 JUNG ON THE SUITABILITY OF YOGA FOR THE WEST

A Critique
In the Light of Sri Aurobindo's Thought

C. G. Jung expressed a good deal of admiration for the various Eastern spiritual ways of life which he generically referred to as yoga, because he saw in their enthronement of intuition a corrective to the paramountcy of the "tyrannical intellect" and the virtual banishment of intuition which he witnessed in the West.[1] Presumably referring to the most widely known system of yoga — Patanjali's Raja Yoga — he wrote that he regarded "this spiritual achievement of the East as one of the greatest things the human mind has ever created".[2] However, Jung was of the firm opinion that the practice of yoga is not suitable for the Westerner.

> The spiritual development of the West has been along entirely different lines from that of the East and has therefore produced conditions which are the most unfavorable soil one can think of for the application of yoga.[3]
>
> I say to whomsoever I can: "Study yoga — you will learn an infinite amount from it — but do not try to apply it, for we Europeans are not so constituted that we apply these methods correctly, just like that".[4]

One reason why Jung regarded the Easterner and the Westerner as constituted differently is related to his theory of the archetypes and their influence on the natural course of religious development. According to this theory, religion in its primitive beginnings takes the form of polydaemonism and magical practice, develops into polytheism and, after passing through several stages, culminates in a religion based on a philosophical view of man and the universe; it is within this last form of religion that a method of self-realization such as yoga develops. Jung states that whereas such a course has fully evolved in the East during its long history, it is not so with the West.[5]

> For what has issued from the Eastern spirit is based upon the peculiar history of that mentality, which is most fundamentally different from ours. Those peoples have experienced an unbroken development from the primitive condition of natural polydaemonism to polytheism in grandest unfoldment and then beyond that to the religion of ideas, within which the original magical practice was able to develop into a method of self-improvement. These assumptions are not applicable to us.[6]

Jung's theory of the natural course of religious development is disaffirmed by what Sri Aurobindo states regarding polytheism in India:

> Indian polytheism is not the popular polytheism of ancient Europe; for here the worshipper of many gods still knows that all his divinities are forms, names, personalities and powers of the One; his gods proceed from the one Purusha*, his goddesses are energies of the one divine Force.[7]

> This explanation of Indian polytheism is not a modern invention to meet Western reproaches; it is to be found explicitly stated in the Gita; it is, still earlier, the sense of the Upanishads; it was clearly stated in so many words in the first ancient days by the "primitive" poets (in truth the profound mystics) of the Veda.[8]

Secondly, what Jung describes as "polydaemonism" and "magical practice" associated with it pertain to occultism, a field which Sri Aurobindo distinguishes from religion:

> There are four main lines which Nature has followed in her attempt to open up the inner being, — religion, occultism, spiritual thought and an inner spiritual realisation and experience....[9]

* Conscious Being.

Occultism is the knowledge and right use of the hidden forces of Nature.[10] These... occult processes... are vulgarly regarded as magic.[11]

The deepest heart, the inmost essence of religion, apart from its outward machinery of creed, cult, ceremony and symbol, is the search for God and the finding of God.[12]

Thus, from Sri Aurobindo's standpoint, Jung's view regarding the difference between the Westerner and the Easterner due to the different evolutionary course of religion in the two hemispheres is based on a misunderstanding of the nature of Eastern religion.

Another reason why Jung regarded yoga as unsuitable for the West lies in his view that the Westerner and the Easterner differ fundamentally in their temperament and mental outlook. Due to this difference, the West cannot graft the intuitive concepts of Eastern yoga on to its scientific mind and ought not to imitate spiritual practices which are alien to the Westerner's own nature.

They [spiritual conditions created by a long tradition] thus create a psychological disposition which makes possible intuitions that transcend consciousness. The Indian mentality has no difficulty in operating intelligently with a concept like *prāṇa*. The West, on the contrary, with its bad habit of wanting to believe on the one hand, and its highly developed scientific and philosophical critique on the other, finds itself in a real dilemma. Either it falls into the trap of faith* and swallows concepts like *prāṇa*, *ātman*, *chakra*, *samādhi*, etc., without giving them a second thought, or its scientific critique repudiates them one and all as "pure mysticism".[13]

Therefore it is sad indeed when the European departs from his own nature and imitates the East or "affects" it in any way. The possibilities open to him would be so much greater if he would

* From Sri Aurobindo's viewpoint, faith, far from being a "trap", is a fundamental requirement for following any spiritual discipline, though a certain degree of scepticism can co-exist with faith.

remain true to himself and evolve out of his own nature all that the East has brought forth in the course of millennia.[14]

Jung's above-stated view appears to be untenable from what Sri Aurobindo wrote to a Western disciple who had come to the conclusion that yoga is impossible for a non-oriental nature due to the different temperament and outlook of the occidental.

> I cannot see any ground for such a conclusion [of the impossibility of the yoga for a non-oriental nature]; it is contrary to all experience. Europeans throughout the centuries have practised with success spiritual disciplines which were akin to oriental yoga and have followed, too, the ways of the inner life which came to them from the East. Their non-oriental nature did not stand in the way. The approach and experiences of Plotinus and the European mystics who derived from him were identical... with the approach and experiences of one type of Indian yoga. Especially, since the introduction of Christianity, Europeans have followed its mystic disciplines which were one in essence with those of Asia, however much they may have differed in forms, names and symbols. If the question be of Indian yoga itself in its own characteristic forms, here too the supposed inability is contradicted by experience. In early times Greeks and Scythians from the West as well as Chinese and Japanese and Cambodians from the East followed without difficulty Buddhist or Hindu disciplines; at the present day an increasing number of occidentals have taken to Vedantic or Vaishnava or other Indian spiritual practices and this objection of incapacity or unsuitableness has never been made either from the side of the disciples or from the side of the Masters.[15]

In response to the disciple's argument that the ability of many Westerners to practise Indian yoga may be explicable by the fact that such Westerners have a Hindu temperament in a Western body, Sri Aurobindo states:

> My own experience contradicts entirely your explanation. I

knew very well Sister Nivedita... and met Sister Christine, — the two closest European disciples of Vivekananda. Both were Westerners to the core and had nothing at all of the Hindu outlook; although Sister Nivedita, an Irish woman, had the power of penetrating by intense sympathy into the ways of life of the people around her, her own nature remained non-oriental to the end. Yet she found no difficulty in arriving at realisation on the lines of Vedanta. Here in the Ashram* I have found the members of it who came from the West (I include especially those who have been here longest) typically occidental with all the quality and also all the difficulties of the Western mind and temperament and they have had to cope with their difficulties, just as the Indian members have been obliged to struggle with the limitations and obstacles created by their temperament and training. No doubt, they have accepted in principle the conditions of the yoga, but they had no Hindu outlook when they came and I do not think they have tried to acquire one. Why should they do so? It is not the Hindu outlook or the Western that fundamentally matters in yoga, but the psychic† turn and the spiritual urge, and these are the same everywhere.[16]

Another characteristic of yoga which, according to Jung, makes its practice impracticable for the Westerner is the requirement of complete trust in the Master and full surrender to him on the part of the disciple. Speaking about Zen Buddhism, Jung asks: "Who among us would place such implicit trust in a superior Master and his incomprehensible ways? This respect for the greater human personality is found only in the East."[17]

The various difficulties encountered in yoga, including the difficulty of surrender, states Sri Aurobindo, afflict both the Indian

* Sri Aurobindo Ashram, Pondicherry, India.
† In common usage the term "psychic" connotes that which is mental or psychological as opposed to physical; in Sri Aurobindo's terminology, the term connotes the soul. Here, used as an adjective, "psychic" means that which pertains to the soul.

and the Westerner, though in different measures, and are by no means insuperable.

The Indian sadhak* has his own difficulties in his approach to the yoga — at least this yoga† — which a Westerner has in less measure. Those of the occidental nature are born of the dominant trend of the European mind in the immediate past. A greater readiness of essential doubt and sceptical reserve; a habit of mental activity as a necessity of nature which makes it more difficult to achieve a complete mental silence; a stronger turn towards outside things born of the plenitude of active life (while the Indian commonly suffers from defects born rather of a depressed or suppressed vital force); a habit of mental and vital self-assertion and sometimes an aggressively vigilant independence which renders difficult any completeness of internal surrender even to a greater Light and Knowledge, even to the divine Influence — these are frequent obstacles. But these things are not universal in Westerners, and they are, on the other hand, present in many Indian sadhaks; they are like the difficulties of the typical Indian nature, superstructural formations, not the very grain of the being. They cannot permanently stand in the way of the soul, if the soul's aspiration is strong and firm, if the spiritual aim is the chief thing in the life.[18]

Yet another reason why Jung regarded yoga to be unsuitable for the West is that, according to him, "Yoga technique applies itself exclusively to the conscious mind and will"[19] and would therefore tend to reinforce the conscious will which is already over-developed in the Westerner. What the Westerner needs, says Jung, is an approach, such as his own method of Active Imagination, that would help him relax the control of the conscious mind, "thus giving the unconscious contents a chance to develop."[20]

...I do not apply yoga methods in principle, because, in the West, nothing ought to be forced on the unconscious. Usually,

---

* Practitioner of yoga.

† Sri Aurobindo's Integral Yoga.

Jung on the Suitability of Yoga for the West 91

consciousness is characterized by an intensity and narrowness that have a cramping effect, and this ought not to be emphasized still further. On the contrary, everything must be done to help the unconscious to reach the conscious mind and to free it from its rigidity.[21]

From Sri Aurobindo's standpoint, Jung's view regarding the unsuitability of yoga for the Westerner because of its "cramping effect" is open to two criticisms:

(1) Sri Aurobindo distinguishes two broad methods of spiritual practice — one of Tapasya or personal effort, consisting of the application of one's conscious will for achieving the goals of the spiritual discipline, the other of surrender, consisting in giving up the ego and opening oneself to the action of a force higher than that of one's personal self.[22] The various spiritual disciplines differ widely in the degree to which their practice involves the two methods. Therefore Jung's statement (perhaps made specifically in regard to Patanjali's system of yoga) that "yoga technique applies itself exclusively to the conscious mind and will" is not applicable to all the numerous and extremely diverse systems of yogic disciplines prevalent in the East.

(2) Regarding personal effort through the exercise of one's conscious will, Sri Aurobindo writes: "Yoga is an endeavour, a tapasya — it can cease to be so only when one surrenders sincerely to a Higher Action and keeps the surrender and makes it complete."[23] But "complete surrender means to cut the knot of the ego in each part of the being."[24] Therefore, as long as the ego is still in command, the exercise of the conscious will is indispensable for purifying the nature and overcoming the ego*.

A salient reason why Jung felt "critically averse"[25] to yoga lies in his view of Samadhi, the eighth stage and culmination of Patanjali's Eightfold Yoga.

---

* From Sri Aurobindo's viewpoint purification or cleansing of the lower nature by the use of conscious will is an essential element of any spiritual discipline — a factor which Jung does not seem to take into account.

> ...*samadhi*, a state of ecstasy,... so far as we know is equivalent to a state of unconsciousness. It makes no difference whether they [yogis] call our unconscious a "universal consciousness"; the fact remains that in their case the unconscious has swallowed up ego-consciousness.[26]

Jung's view of Samadhi as a state of unconsciousness is based on the common meaning of Samadhi as a state of yogic trance. This is obvious from Jung's description of Samadhi as "'withdrawnness', i.e., a condition in which all connections with the world are absorbed into the inner world."[27] That is how Samadhi is conceived in some of the yogic disciplines, such as Patanjali's Raja Yoga. But, as Sri Aurobindo points out, "the word [Samadhi] is capable, as in the Gita, of a much wider sense."[28]

> The sign of the man in Samadhi is not that he loses consciousness of objects and surroundings and of his mental and physical self and cannot be recalled to it even by burning or torture of the body, — the ordinary idea of the matter; trance is a particular intensity, not the essential sign. The test is the expulsion of all desires, their inability to get at the mind, and it is the inner state from which this freedom arises, the delight of the soul gathered within itself with the mind equal and still and high-poised above the attractions and repulsions, the alternations of sunshine and storm and stress of the external life. It is drawn inward even when acting outwardly; it is concentrated in self even when gazing out upon things; it is directed wholly to the Divine even when to the outward vision of others busy and preoccupied with the affairs of the world.[29]
>
> It is this calm, desireless, griefless fixity of the Buddhi* in self-poise and self-knowledge to which the Gita gives the name of Samadhi.[30]

Stating the meaning of Samadhi in his own yoga, Sri Aurobindo writes:

---

* The discriminating principle which is at once intelligence and will.

Jung on the Suitability of Yoga for the West

> ...a certain self-gathered state of our whole existence lifted into that superconscient truth, unity and infinity of self-aware, self-blissful existence... that is the meaning we shall give to the term Samadhi. Not merely a state withdrawn from all consciousness of the outward, withdrawn even from all consciousness of the inward into what exists beyond both... but a settled existence in the Chit* and Infinite, united and identified with it....[31]

Therefore Jung's criticism of yoga related to its goal of Samadhi as a trance state would apply only to those forms of yoga which aim at the yogic trance as the ultimate goal; it does not apply to the yogic disciplines which aim at "waking Samadhi".

Even as a state of yogic trance, Samadhi can be described as an unconscious state only from the viewpoint of the ordinary waking or mental consciousness — that which Jung regards as consciousness. From the viewpoint of yoga, which speaks of various levels of consciousness — of which mental consciousness is the most superficial level — Samadhi, far from being unconsciousness, is a state "in which the consciousness goes inside"[32] and "in which one enters into a massed consciousness containing in it all the powers of being but all compressed within itself and concentrated solely on itself...a state admitting us into the higher planes of the spirit normally now superconscient to our waking being."[33]

Thus the yogic trance which, from Jung's *theoretical* viewpoint, represents a lapse into unconsciousness, is from the yogic *experiential* viewpoint a plunge into a greater consciousness.

Conclusion

Jung's views of yoga were apparently derived chiefly from Patanjali's Yoga Sutras on which he wrote a detailed commenatry. These views were unduly generalised and applied to all other Eastern systems of spiritual discipline. Some of Jung's views regarding the unsuitability of yoga for Westerners

---

* Consciousness.

stem from his general theories. Thus his view that the Easterner and the Westerner are constituted differently because of the difference in the historical development of religion in the East and the West is based on his questionable theory of the way in which the natural course of religious development is shaped by the archetypes. Similarly his view that Samadhi is a state of unconsciousness is related to his untenable theory that consciousness cannot exist without the ego. As general statements applied to all Eastern systems of spiritual discipline, the various reasons given by Jung for considering yoga unsuitable for the West are seen to be unsound from the viewpoint of Sri Aurobindo's thought and experience.

REFERENCES

1. C. G. Jung, *Alchemical Studies*, Collected Works, Vol. 13 (Bollingen Series XX, Pantheon Books, 1958), p. 9.
2. C. G. Jung, *Psychology and Religion: West and East*, Collected Works, Vol. 11, p. 537.
3. Ibid.
4. Ibid., p. 534.
5. J. Borelli, "Jung's Criticism of Yoga Spirituality" in Harold Coward, *Jung and Eastern Thought* (Albany: State University of New York Press, 1985), p. 83.
6. C. G. Jung, quoted in J. Borelli, "Jung's Criticism of Yoga Spirituality" in *Jung and Eastern Thought*, p. 84.
7. Sri Aurobindo, *The Foundations of Indian Culture*, Sri Aurobindo Birth Centenary Library (hereafter SABCL) (Pondicherry: Sri Aurobindo Ashram, 1970-1975), Vol. 14, p. 135.
8. Ibid., p. 137.
9. Sri Aurobindo, *The Life Divine*, SABCL, Vol. 19, p. 860.
10. Sri Aurobindo, *Letters on Yoga*, SABCL, Vol. 22, p. 75.
11. Ibid., p. 214.
12. Sri Aurobindo, *Social and Political Thought*, SABCL, Vol. 15, p. 122.
13. C. G. Jung, *Psychology and Religion: West and East*, p. 533.
14. C. G. Jung, *Alchemical Studies*, pp. 9-10.
15. Sri Aurobindo, *Letters on Yoga*, SABCL, Vol. 23, pp. 555-56.
16. Ibid., p. 557.
17. C. G. Jung, *Psychology and Religion: West and East*, p. 533.
18. Sri Aurobindo, *Letters on Yoga*, SABCL, Vol. 23, pp. 558-59.

19. C. G. Jung, *Psychology and Religion: West and East*, p. 535.
20. Ibid., p. 537.
21. Ibid.
22. Sri Aurobindo, *Letters on Yoga*, SABCL, Vol. 23, pp. 586-88.
23. Ibid., p. 612.
24. Ibid., p. 591.
25. C. G. Jung, *Psychology and Religion: West and East*, p. 537.
26. C. G. Jung, *The Archetypes and the Collective Unconscious*, Collected Works, Vol. 9, Part 1, p. 287.
27. C. G. Jung, *Psychology and Religion: West and East*, p. 562.
28. Sri Aurobindo, *The Synthesis of Yoga*, SABCL, Vol. 20, p. 305.
29. Sri Aurobindo, *Essays on the Gita*, SABCL, Vol. 13, pp. 94-95.
30. Ibid., p. 94.
31. Sri Aurobindo, *The Synthesis of Yoga*, SABCL, Vol. 20, p. 307.
32. Sri Aurobindo, *Letters on Yoga*, SABCL, Vol. 23, p. 1014.
33. Sri Aurobindo, *The Life Divine*, SABCL, Vol. 18, p. 452 fn.

7 PSYCHOLOGICAL DISTURBANCES

A Model Based on Sri Aurobindo's Yoga Psychology

...not a single person is normal, because to be normal is to be divine.[1]

THE MOTHER

Since, as Sri Aurobindo has stated, "Yoga is nothing but practical psychology",[2] resolving the psychological problems inherent in human nature is the crux of the practice of yoga. As such, yoga necessarily deals with psychological disturbances — the subject-matter of clinical psychology and psychiatry. The purpose of this essay is to explain the nature of psychological disturbances from the viewpoint of Sri Aurobindo's psychological thought implicit in his Integral Yoga. In doing so, we will draw mostly from specific references in the writings of Sri Aurobindo and the Mother bearing on the subject.

An understanding of the nature of psychological disturbances from the standpoint of Integral Yoga may be approached from the description of the state of psychological health contained in the following message given by the Mother for newcomers to Sri Aurobindo International University Centre (now called Sri Aurobindo International Centre of Education):

> Some of them come with a mental aspiration, either to serve or to learn; others come in the hope of doing yoga, of finding the Divine and uniting with Him; finally there are those who want to devote themselves entirely to the divine work upon earth. All of them come impelled by their psychic being, which wants to lead them towards self-realisation. They come with their psychic in front and ruling their consciousness; they have a psychic contact with people and things. Everything seems beautiful and good to them, their health improves, their

consciousness grows more luminous; they feel happy, peaceful and safe; they think that they have reached their utmost possibility of consciousness. This peace and fullness and joy given by the psychic contact they naturally find everywhere, in everything and everybody. It gives an openness towards the true consciousness pervading here and working out everything. So long as the openness is there, the peace, the fullness and the joy remain with their immediate results of progress, health and fitness in the physical, quietness and goodwill in the vital, clear understanding and broadness in the mental and a general feeling of security and satisfaction.[3]

Two points may be noted in the above-quoted description of the state of psychological well-being. First, well-being is described in terms of states of the body, the vital and the mind: "...health and fitness in the physical, quietness and goodwill in the vital, clear understanding and broadness in the mental and a general feeling of security and satisfaction." Secondly, such a state of psychological health is ascribed to the fact that the psychic is in front and rules the consciousness, as a result of which there is a psychic contact with people and things.

Before stating the implications of what has just been said, it is necessary to explain some of the less familiar terms used above. Whereas terms such as "mind", "vital", "physical" and "psychic" are not new, they have special meanings in the language of Integral Yoga.

In ordinary usage, "mind" has a rather vague and too broad a connotation: anything that does not clearly pertain to the body is often conceived to be related to the mind. Thus all processes of thinking, feeling and willing (cognition, affect and volition, as they are termed in psychology) are ascribed to the mind. But in the language of Integral Yoga, "mind" refers to that part of the human being which has to do solely with cognitive functions and processes. Feeling or affect is regarded as pertaining to the vital, whereas will or volition can be either mental or vital. Sri Aurobindo clarifies the distinction between the mind and the vital as follows:

The "Mind" in the ordinary use of the word covers indiscriminately the whole consciousness, for man is a mental being and mentalises everything; but in the language of this yoga the words "mind" and "mental" are used to connote specially the part of the nature which has to do with cognition and intelligence, with ideas, with mental or thought perceptions, the reactions of thought to things, with the truly mental movements and formations, mental vision and will, etc., that are part of his intelligence. The vital has to be carefully distinguished from mind, even though it has a mind element transfused into it; the vital is the Life-nature made up of desires, sensations, feelings, passions, energies of action, will of desire, reactions of the desire-soul in man and of all that play of possessive and other related instincts, anger, fear, greed, lust, etc., that belong to this field of the nature. Mind and vital are mixed up on the surface of the consciousness, but they are quite separate forces in themselves and as soon as one gets behind the ordinary surface consciousness one sees them as separate, discovers their distinction and can with the aid of this knowledge analyse their surface mixtures.[4]

Another equally important concept is that of the physical being, which is considered not merely as the gross body, but as something that has a distinct consciousness of its own which is different from that of mind and vital, though interfused with mental and vital consciousness. As Sri Aurobindo explains:

Each plane of our being — mental, vital, physical — has its own consciousness, separate though interconnected and interacting; but to our outer mind and sense, in our waking experience, they are all confused together. The body, for instance, has its own consciousness and acts from it, even without any mental will of our own or even against that will, and our surface mind knows very little about this body-consciousness, feels it only in an imperfect way, sees only its results and has the greatest difficulty in finding out their causes.[5]

Some of the chief characteristics of physical consciousness are inertia, obscurity, mechanical activity, repetitiveness, chaotic movement and narrowness or constriction. Unlike the mental and the vital planes of the being which are relatively more conscious, the physical plane is largely below the level of awareness. Therefore we become better aware of the characteristics of physical consciousness when these manifest through the "physical mind" (part of the mind interfused with physical consciousness) or through the "physical vital" (part of the vital which is interfused with physical consciousness). The terms "physical mind" and "physical vital" will become clearer when we describe the psychological disturbances pertaining to these parts of the being.

The term "psychic" is used in Integral Yoga to refer to the inmost part of the being which supports the outer nature of body, vital and mind and which, in most human beings, is hidden and veiled by the activities of physical, vital and mental consciousness.

The reason for dwelling at some length on definitions of the mental, the vital and the physical lies in the fact that in Integral Yoga, psychological disturbances are seen as springing from various *inherent* characteristics of physical, vital and mental consciousness and of their subdivisions made up of their intermixtures. Specific kinds of disturbances are associated with each of these parts of the being as indicated below.

Disturbances Associated with the Mind

From one viewpoint, the basic cause of all psychological disturbances lies in the nature of the mind. The peculiar characteristic of mental consciousness is that it is self-reflective, that is, it can objectivise itself. One part of the mind can separate itself and observe the rest as an object. The part that stands back serves as a mirror which reflects to the observing mind its own state. This objectivising nature of the mind accounts for the very awareness of psychological disturbances. Secondly, the agony of any disturbance is magnified by several other factors related to the mind, such as memory, anticipation, imagination and the mind's inherent need — in the face of its essential incapacity — to understand and find a solution to the problems causing the disturbances. What has just been stated about the constitutional nature of the mind in its relationship to psychological disturbances is largely a paraphrase of the following remarks made by the Mother:

> It is obvious that what especially characterises man is this mental capacity of watching himself live. The animal lives spontaneously, automatically, and if it watches itself live, it must be to a very minute and insignificant degree, and that is why it is peaceful and does not worry. Even if an animal is suffering because of an accident or an illness, this suffering is reduced to a minimum by the fact that it does not observe it, does not project it in its consciousness and into the future, does not imagine things about its illness or its accident.
>
> With man there has begun this perpetual worrying about what is going to happen, and this worry is the principal, if not the sole cause of his torment. With this objectivising consciousness there has begun anxiety, painful imaginations, worry, torment, anticipation of future catastrophes, with the result that most men — and not the least conscious, the most conscious — live in perpetual torment. Man is too conscious to be indifferent, he is not conscious enough to know what will happen. Truly it could be said without fear of making a mistake that of all earth's creatures he is the most miserable. The human being is used to being like that because it is an atavistic state which he has inherited from his ancestors, but it is truly a miserable condition. And it is only with this spiritual capacity of rising to a higher level and replacing the animal's unconsciousness by a spiritual super-consciousness that there comes into the being not only the capacity to see the goal of existence and to foresee the culmination of the effort but also a clear-sighted trust in a higher spiritual power to which one can surrender one's whole being, entrust oneself, give the responsibility for one's life and future and so abandon all worries.

Of course, it is impossible for man to fall back to the level of the animal and lose the consciousness he has acquired; therefore, for him there is only one means, one way to get out of this condition he is in, which I call a miserable one, and to emerge into a higher state where worry is replaced by a trusting surrender and the certitude of a luminous culmination — this way is to change the consciousness.

Truly speaking there is no condition more miserable than being responsible for an existence to which one doesn't have the key, that is, of which one doesn't have the threads that can guide and solve the problems. The animal sets itself no problems: it just lives. Its instinct drives it, it relies on a collective consciousness which has an innate knowledge and is higher than itself, but it is automatic, spontaneous, it has no need to will something and make an effort to bring it about, it is quite naturally like that, and as it is not responsible for its life, it does not worry. With man is born the sense of having to depend on himself, and as he does not have the necessary knowledge the result is a perpetual torment. This torment can come to an end only with a total surrender to a higher consciousness than his own to which he can totally entrust himself, hand over his worries and leave the care of guiding his life and organising everything.

How can a problem be solved when one doesn't have the necessary knowledge? And the unfortunate thing is that man believes that he has to resolve all the problems of his life, and he does not have the knowledge needed to do it. That is the source, the origin of all his troubles — that perpetual question, "What should I do?" which is followed by another one still more acute, "What is going to happen?" and at the same time, more or less, the inability to answer.[6]

Whereas simple awareness through objectivisation belongs to the mind proper, the fearful imaginations and anticipations, resulting in anxiety, come from the part of the mind intermixed with the vital, called the vital mind.

Another manifestation of the vital mind in relation to psychological disturbances is to be seen in the so-called "defence mechanisms" associated with all psychiatric disorders. A defence mechanism is defined as an unconscious process which serves to ward off a painful feeling, such as anxiety, guilt, etc., from the level of awareness. One of the chief defence mechanisms is rationalization, by which the mind colludes with the vital in providing specious explanations and justifications for impulses and desires of the vital. As Sri Aurobindo states:

> The vital started in its evolution with obedience to impulse and no reason — as for strategy, the only strategy it understands is some tactics by which it can compass its desires. It does not like the voice of knowledge and wisdom — but curiously enough by the necessity which has grown up in man of justifying action by reason, the *vital mind* has developed a strategy of its own which is to get the reason to find out reasons for justifying its own feelings and impulses.[7]

Another example of a defence mechanism is that of projection, by which we tend to attribute a feeling or motive to another person who, in fact, does not have that feeling or motive. Such a phenomenon is due to the fact that the cognitive functions of perception and judgment are, in most human beings, strongly influenced by the feelings and impulses of the vital. As the Mother observes:

> The sense organs are under the influence of the psychological state of the individual because something comes in between the eye's perception and the brain's reception. It is very subtle; the brain receives the eye's perceptions through the nerves; there is no reasoning, it is so to say instantaneous, but there is a short passage between the eye's perception and the cell which is to respond and evaluate it in the brain. And it is this evaluation of the brain which is under the influence of feelings. It is the small vibration between what the eye sees and what the brain estimates which often falsifies the response. And it is not a question of good faith, for even the most sincere persons do

not know what is happening, even very calm people, without any violent emotion, who do not even feel an emotion, are influenced in this way without being aware of the intervention of this little falsifying vibration.

It is only when you have conquered all attraction and all repulsion that you can have a correct judgment. As long as there are things that attract you and things that repel you, it is not possible for you to have an absolutely sure functioning of the senses.[8]

What is called a projection in psychopathology is simply an exaggeration of the everyday distortion of our perceptions and judgments by the vital mind alluded to in the above-quoted passage.

Less obvious forms of disturbances attributable to the mind are related to the part of the mind that is intermixed with the physical consciousness, called the physical mind. The mechanical and chaotic activity of physical consciousness, mentioned previously, is reflected in the ceaseless and incoherent thought activity which turns the mind into a veritable market-place where thoughts constantly come and go in a disorderly manner.

Related to the chaotic nature of the physical mind are its features of unsteadiness and susceptibility to the influence of the things in the physical environment which determine to a large extent the way most people think. Referring to this susceptibility to the external determinants of ordinary thinking, the Mother remarks:

One believes that he has his own way of thinking. Not at all. It depends totally upon the people one speaks with or the books he has read or on the mood he is in. It depends also on whether you have a good or bad digestion, it depends on whether you are shut up in a room without proper ventilation or whether you are in the open air; it depends on whether you have a beautiful landscape before you; it depends on whether there is sunshine or rain! You are not aware of it, but you think all kind of things, completely different according to a heap of things which have nothing to do with you![9]

Most people, who are not aware of the chaotic activity of the physical mind and its unsteadiness, do not experience these characteristics of the mind as disturbances. It is only when one takes up a discipline for quieting or controlling the mind that one becomes conscious of these deeply ingrained disturbances of the mind.

Another characteristic of the physical consciousness, also mentioned previously, is its mechanical repetitiveness. This trait is manifested in the automatic recurrences of thoughts and words to which the physical mind is prone. The Mother gives a familiar example of this feature of the physical mind:

> For example, you see, if it fancies counting: "One, two, three, four", then it will go on: "One, two, three, four; one, two, three, four." And you may think of all kinds of things, but it goes on: "One, two, three, four", like that... (*Mother laughs*). Or it catches hold of three words, four words and repeats them and goes on repeating them; and unless one turns away with a certain violence and punches it soundly, telling it, "Keep quiet!", it continues in this way, indefinitely.*[10]

Again, most people are either not aware or not disturbed by such repetitive thoughts unless the thoughts are of an upsetting nature, such as guilt-laden, hostile or lewd thoughts which assume an obsessive form so that one is unable to stop them.

Still another psychological disturbance related to the physical mind stems from the obscurity of the physical consciousness, leading to perpetual doubt. Here too, though the disturbance is inherent in the very nature of the physical mind, one usually becomes aware of it only when the disturbance is pronounced and manifests in compulsive behaviour, such as the compulsion to check and recheck if a door has been locked or if the gas has been turned off.

---

* It is interesting to note the similarity between the method recommended here by the Mother for quieting the physical mind and the technique of "thought-stopping" employed in modern behavioural therapies in which the therapist, on observing an undesirable thought process in a client, shouts "Stop!" The client is then instructed on using this technique for stopping unproductive or counterproductive ways of thinking as soon as they are detected.

Psychological Disturbances

In response to the question why one doubts something that one knows to be true, the Mother narrates a personal experience to illustrate the obscurity of the physical mind:

> ...the truth is that the physical mind is truly completely stupid! You can prove it very easily. It is constructed probably as a kind of control, and in order to make sure that things are done as they ought to be. I think that this is its normal work.... But it has made it a habit to doubt everything.
>
> I think I have already told you about the small experiment I made one day. I removed my control and left the control to the physical mind — it is the physical mind which doubts. So I made the following experiment: I went into a room, then came out of the room and closed the door. I had decided to close the door; and when I came to another room this mind, the material mind, the physical mind, you see, said, "Are you sure you have locked the door?" Now, I did not control, you know... I said, "Very well, I obey it!" I went back to see. I observed that the door was closed. I came back. As soon as I couldn't see the door any longer, it told me, "Have you verified properly?" So I went back again.... And this went on till I decided: "Come now, that's enough, isn't it? closed or not, I am not going back any more to see!" This could have gone on the whole day. It is made like that. It stops being like that only when a higher mind, the rational mind, tells it, "Keep quiet!" Otherwise it goes on indefinitely.... So, if by ill-luck you are centred there, in this mind, even the things you know higher up as quite true, even things of which you have a physical proof — like that of the closed door, it doubts, it will doubt, because it is built of doubt.[11]

One form of doubt that plagues the physical mind is indecision when faced with several desires pulling from different directions. When such an indecision takes an extreme form, paralyzing the action, it is recognized as a pathological symptom, referred to as abulia. However, in its milder form, indecision is a normal characteristic in all those who have a somewhat active physical mind. Regarding the dynamics of indecision, Sri Aurobindo observes: "Those who can't choose, have the vital indecision and it is usually due to a too active physical mind, seeing too many things or too many ideas at a time."[12]

From what has been stated above regarding the disturbances of the physical mind, it should be apparent that the obsessive-compulsive neurosis — characterized by obsessive thoughts, compulsive behaviour, indecision, etc. — is related chiefly to the physical mind.

Disturbances Associated with the Vital

The vital, like the mind, has certain inherent disturbances. In the first place, the vital, as the source of desires, longings and cravings, constitutes a disturbance in itself, though not felt as such except by very few. The nature of desire as a form of suffering is well brought out in the following remarks made by the Mother in response to the question: Where does desire come from?

> The Buddha said that it comes from ignorance. It is more or less that. It is something in the being which fancies that it needs something else in order to be satisfied. And the proof that it is ignorance is that when one has satisfied it, one no longer cares for it, at least ninety-nine and a half times out of a hundred....
> Take for instance... you see something which is — which seems to you or is — very beautiful, very harmonious, very pleasant; if you have the true consciousness, you experience this joy of seeing, of being in a conscious contact with something very beautiful, very harmonious, and then that's all. It stops there. You have the joy of it — that such a thing exists, you see. And this is quite common among artists who have a sense of beauty. For example, an artist may see a beautiful creature and have the joy of observing the beauty, grace, harmony of movement and all that, and that's all. It stops there. He is perfectly happy, perfectly satisfied, because he has seen

something beautiful. An ordinary consciousness — altogether ordinary, dull like all ordinary consciousness — as soon as it sees something beautiful, whether it be an object or a person, hop! "I want it!" It is deplorable, you know. And into the bargain it doesn't even have the joy of the beauty, because it has the anguish of desire. It misses that and has nothing in exchange, because there is nothing pleasant in desiring anything. It only puts you in an unpleasant state, that's all.[13]

The chief point to be noted in the above-quoted passage is that the "anguish of desire" constitutes an inherent disturbance of the vital. As long as the vital consciousness prevails, one is in "an unpleasant state" of desiring, and it is impossible to have inner peace.

Besides desire, the vital is the spring of a host of other disturbing feelings. One of the chief vital disturbances is fear. As a rule, human beings are constantly subject to fear, though very few are aware of the continual undercurrent of fear. As the Mother observes:

The normal human condition is a state filled with apprehensions and fears; if you observe your mind deeply for ten minutes, you will find that for nine out of ten it is full of fears — it carries in it fear about many things, big and small, near and far, seen and unseen, and though you do not usually take conscious notice of it, it is there all the same.[14]

It is not surprising, therefore, that anxiety, which is simply "fear spread thin", is the commonest of all psychiatric symptoms.

Closely related to fear are two other major disturbances of the

---

* It has been observed that a depressed patient can often be brought out of depression by making the patient angry. This might lead one to think that the opposite of depression is anger. However, from the viewpoint of yoga psychology, depression is a *state* rather than an emotion. The opposite state is that of revolt, which may be associated with various emotions, such as anger, resentment and vengefulness.

vital, namely, anger and depression. About these two feelings the Mother says:

> ...one is almost constantly in an ordinary vital state where the least unpleasant thing very spontaneously and easily brings you depression — depression if you are a weak person, revolt if you are a strong one.* Every desire which is not satisfied, every impulse which meets an obstacle, every unpleasant contact with outside things, very easily and very spontaneously creates depression or revolt, for that is the normal state of things.[15]

Besides the three emotional factors just mentioned, there are many others which produce psychological disturbances. One particular feeling which may be mentioned because of its wide prevalence in modern civilization is impatience. Since a desire, unless checked by the mental will or by another counteracting desire, has an innate drive to satsify itself immediately, impatience may be said to be an essential characteristic of the vital. And the stronger the desires, the greater the impatience. This tendency of the vital is at the basis of the present-day "time urgency" which has been identified as one of the chief traits that characterize what Friedman and Rosenman have labelled Type A behaviour, regarded by these researchers in the field of cardiology as the chief factor in coronary artery and heart disease and high blood pressure.[16] The Mother alludes to this "hurry sickness" in the following passage:

> We — I mean men — live harassed lives. It is a kind of half-awareness of the shortness of their lives; they do not think of it, but they feel it half-consciously. And so they are always wanting — quick, quick, quick — to rush from one thing to another, to do one thing quickly and move on to the next one, instead of letting each thing live in its own eternity. They are always wanting: forward, forward, forward.... And the work is spoilt.
>
> That is why some people have preached: the only moment that matters is the present moment. In practice it is not true,

but from the psychological point of view it ought to be true. That is to say, to live to the utmost of one's capacities at every minute, without planning or wanting, waiting or preparing for the next. Because you are always hurrying, hurrying, hurrying... nothing you do is good. You are in a state of inner tension which is completely false — completely false.

All those who have tried to be wise have always said it — the Chinese preached it, the Indians preached it — to live in the awareness of Eternity. In Europe also they said that one should contemplate the sky and the stars and identify oneself with their infinitude — all things that widen you and give you peace.

These are means, but they are indispensable.

And I have observed this in the cells of the body; they always seem to be in a hurry to do what they have to do, lest they have no time to do it. So they do nothing properly. Muddled people — some people turn everything upside down, their movements are jerky and confused — have this to a high degree, this kind of haste — quick, quick, quick.... Yesterday, someone was complaining of rheumatic pains and he was saying, "Oh, it is such a waste of time. I do things so slowly!" I said (*Mother smiles*), "So what!" He didn't like it. You see, for someone to complain when he is in pain means that he is soft, that is all; but to say, "I am wasting so much time, I do things so slowly!" It gave a very clear picture of the haste in which men live. You go hurtling through life... to go where?... You end with a crash![17]

It is not only the unpleasant feelings such as those discussed above that cause disturbance. The excitement produced by pleasant feelings also leads to a definite psychophysiological disturbance. An interesting corroboration of this fact is provided by two medical researchers, Holmes and Rahe, who have developed the Life Change Index — an inventory that gives statistical values to various common life events with regard to the degree of stress each type of event produces in an average person. The inventory includes not only such unhappy incidents as the death of a spouse, being fired from a job, etc., but also happy events such as marriage, outstanding personal achievements, etc. It is interesting that the inventory gives a higher stress production value to a vacation and to Christmas than to being convicted of minor violations of the law! Holmes and Rahe attribute the stress caused by various life events to the adaptation that a person is called upon to make in response to the changes produced by an event. However, from the viewpoint of yoga psychology, the underlying factor which disturbs the homeostatic equilibrium is the emotional reaction evoked by an event.

These findings in the field of medical research corroborate the view of Integral Yoga that suffering being inherent in the very nature of the untransformed vital, even what is experienced as a pleasant excitation of the vital leads to disturbances.

The fact that repression of the vital leads to disturbances is well-recognized both in psychiatry and yoga, and therefore need not be elaborated here. What is not recognized in psychiatry is that the free expression of the vital, too, produces disturbances. Even though most psychiatrists would recommend moderation in the satisfaction of desires, such a recommendation is based upon commonsense and physiological considerations rather than on psychiatric principles. For psychiatry speaks of no specific psychological disturbances resulting from an excessive satisfaction of desires. And as for the normal expression of desires, this is deemed not only perfectly all right but indispensable for maintaining psychological health.

Yoga, on the other hand, looks upon desire *per se* as a disturbance. The metapsychology of such a view is expressed in the following words of the Mother:

> To have needs is to assert a weakness; to claim something proves that we lack what we claim. To desire is to be impotent; it is to recognise our limitations and confess our incapacity to overcome them.[18]

As for the free play of desires, yoga holds that "...this brings on fairly serious disorders."[19]

The essential morbidity of the untransformed vital nature is particularly evident in its masochistic tendency to continue clinging to a disturbance and to wallow in it. Sri Aurobindo refers to this trait in a letter:

> ...a habit of the human vital — the tendency to keep any touch of grief, anger, vexation, etc. or any kind of emotional, vital or mental disturbance, to make much of it, to prolong it, not to wish to let it go, to return to it even when the cause of disturbance is past and could be forgotten, always to remember and bring it up when it can. This is a common trait of the human nature and a quite customary movement.[20]

Disturbances Associated with the Physical

The most prominent characteristic of physical consciousness is inertia or Tamas. Therefore an individual with a predominantly physical consciousness is slow in reacting to stimulation. An intense stimulus is needed to produce an emotional reaction in tamasic individuals. As the Mother remarks about such persons:

> ...they always need new excitements, dramas, murders, suicides, etc. to get the impression of something.... And there is nothing, nothing that makes one more wicked and cruel than tamas. For it is this need of excitement which shakes you up a little, makes you come out of yourself.[21]

Because of the inertia of physical consciousness, what is experienced as a pleasant stimulus by the average person is too feeble or dull for the individual whose consciousness is chiefly that of the physical. In order to feel a pleasant stimulation, such a tamasic individual needs a much more intense stimulus, such that an average person would experience as unpleasant or even painful. Such a condition represents a psychological disturbance because it is a form of masochism — a state in which an individual finds pleasurable what is experienced by most people as painful. Thus masochistic disorders are related partly to the physical consciousness.

An aspect of inertia is passivity, which often manifests as a weakness of the will. Sri Aurobindo speaks of this as follows:

> It [the weakness of the will] is a first result of coming down into the physical consciousness or of the physical consciousness coming up prominently.... The physical consciousness is full of inertia — it wants not to move but to be moved by whatever forces and that is its habit.[22]

> The physical consciousness or at least the more external parts of it are ... in their nature inert — obeying whatever force they are habituated to obey, but not acting on their own initiative. When there is a strong influence of the physical inertia or when one is down in this part of the consciousness the mind feels like the material Nature that action of will is impossible.[23]

Weakness of the will may be regarded by some as pertaining to the province of ethics and morality rather than that of psychopathology. However, we must recognize that weakness of the will is a disturbance of volition and as such it is as relevant to psychopathology as disorders of the other two basic psychological functions, namely, thinking and feeling.

What have been called habit disorders in psychiatry are also partly related to the physical consciousness, for the force of habit is derived from the inertia and mechanical responsiveness of physical consciousness. As Sri Aurobindo explains:

> In the physical being the power of past impressions is very great, because it is by the process of repeated impressions that consciousness was made to manifest in matter — and also by the habitual reactions of consciousness to these impressions, what the psychologists, I suppose, would call behaviour.[24]

> The physical is the slave of certain forces which create a habit and drive it through the mechanical power of the habit. So long as the mind gives consent, you do not notice the slavery; but if the mind withdraws its consent, then you feel the servitude, you feel a force pushing you in spite of the mind's will. It is very obstinate and repeats itself till the habit, the inner habit

revealing itself in the outward act, is broken. It is like a machine which once set in motion repeats the same movement.[25]

The part of the physical being which is intermixed with the vital is called the vital-physical. It is the part of the being that governs reactions of the nerves. As the nerves are involved in all psychological disturbances and most physiological ones as well, Sri Aurobindo observes: "It [the vital-physical] is also largely responsible for most of the suffering and disease of mind or body to which the physical being is subject in Nature."[26]

The Subconscient

Not mentioned so far is the plane of consciousness below the physical, called the subconscient. Sri Aurobindo describes this part of the being as follows:

> That part of us which we can strictly call subconscient because it is below the level of mind and conscious life, inferior and obscure, covers the purely physical and vital elements of our constitution of bodily being, unmentalised, unobserved by the mind, uncontrolled by it in their action. It can be held to include the dumb occult consciousness, dynamic but not sensed by us, which operates in the cells and nerves and all the corporeal stuff and adjusts their life process and automatic responses. It covers also those lowest functionings of submerged sense-mind which are more operative in the animal and in plant life.[27]

The psychology of Integral Yoga confirms the modern psychological theory that regards the subconscious as the storehouse of things which have been repressed and which lie buried, but not dead, and which continue to influence powerfully the waking as well as the dreaming state.

The "repetition compulsion", of which Freud spoke, is a well-recognised phenomenon in Integral Yoga which regards it as related to the subconscient. Sri Aurobindo speaks of it in the following excerpts:

> The habit of strong recurrence of the same things in our physical consciousness, so that it is difficult to get rid of its habits, is largely due to a subconscient support. The subconscient is full of irrational habits.[28]

> The subconscient is the main support of all habitual movements, especially the physical and lower vital movements. When something is thrown out of the vital or physical, it very usually goes down into the subconscient and remains there as if in seed and comes up again when it can. That is the reason why it is so difficult to get rid of habitual vital movements or to change the character; for, supported or refreshed from this source, preserved in this matrix your vital movements, even when suppressed or repressed, surge up and recur.[29]

The recurrence of chronic illness is, according to Integral Yoga, a habit of the subconscient.[30]

Sri Aurobindo states that drug addiction, too, is based on a subconscient habit. "It is the habit in the subconscient material* that feels an artificial need created by the past and does not care whether it is harmful or disturbing to the nerves or not. That is the nature of all intoxicants (wine, tobacco, cocaine etc.)...."[31]

More concealed disturbances which are related to the subconscient are the prenatal influences of the parents on the infant. The state of consciousness of the parents at the time of conception is regarded in yoga psychology as a powerful factor that underlies the physical, intellectual and characterological defects and deficiencies which a child may manifest. In response to a question whether the wickedness found in some children is due to the fact that the parents did not wish to have the children, the Mother makes the following statement regarding the subconscient influence of the parents on the new-born:

> It is perhaps a subconscious wickedness in the parents. It is said that people throw out their wickedness from themselves

---

* The subconscient material is the grossest part of the material or physical consciousness which is intermixed with the subconscient.

by giving it birth in their children. One has always a shadow in oneself. There are people who project this outside — that does not always free them from it, but still perhaps it comforts them! But it is the child who "profits" by it, don't you see? It is quite evident that the state of consciousness in which the parents are at the moment [of conception] is of capital importance. If they have very low and vulgar ideas, the children will reflect them quite certainly. And all these children who are ill-formed, ill-bred, incomplete (specially from the point of view of intelligence: with holes, things missing), children who are only half-conscious and half-formed — this is always due to the fault of the state of consciousness in which the parents were when they conceived the child. Even as the state of consciousness of the last moments of life is of capital importance for the future of the one who is departing, so too the state of consciousness in which the parents are at the moment of conception gives a sort of stamp to the child, which it will reflect throughout its life. So, these are apparently such little things — the mood of the moment, the moment's aspiration or degradation, anything whatsoever, everything that takes place at a particular moment — it seems to be so small a thing, and it has so great a consequence: it brings into the world a child who is incomplete or wicked or finally a failure. And people are not aware of that.

Later, when the child behaves nastily, they scold it. But they should begin by scolding themselves, telling themselves: "In what a horrible state of consciousness must I have been when I brought that child into the world". For it is truly that.[32]

Psychosomatic Disorders

Psychosomatic disorders are bodily illnesses which are associated with psychological disturbances. In such illnesses of the

* Such a viewpoint was part of the basis for the classification system adopted by the American Psychiatric Association in the third revision of its *Diagnostic and Statistical Manual* published in 1980.

body, a psychological disturbance such as anxiety, anger, fear, jealousy or the like plays at least a partial role as an exciting or contributory cause. Until quite recently, only certain bodily illnesses, such as asthma, migraine, high blood pressure, etc., were regarded as psychosomatic, though the list has been growing. However, a new viewpoint which has recently emerged holds that the manifestation of *all* bodily disorders is psychological to some degree.* This viewpoint is consonant with what is implied in Sri Aurobindo's previously quoted remark that the vital-physical part of the being is "largely responsible for most of the suffering and disease of mind or body to which the physical being is subject". Yoga psychology traces not only major illnesses but also minor day-to-day variations in the state of one's health to psychological factors. As the Mother observes:

> ...each man can make his own experiment. If one has a bad throat, this may be due to the fact that the day before one was in a state of depression. Or perhaps one is very unhappy, dissatisfied, one finds everything very bad, and the next day one gets a cold in the head.[33]

Furthermore, according to yoga psychology, the specific part of the body affected by illness is a clue to the specific nature of the psychological disturbance associated with the illness. As the Mother states:

> Each spot of the body is symbolical of an inner movement; there is there a world of subtle correspondences.... The particular place in the body affected by an illness is an index to the nature of the inner disharmony that has taken place. It points to the origin, it is a sign of the cause of the ailment.[34]

The following is an example of such a specific correspondence.

> It is particularly noticeable that all the digestive functions are extremely sensitive to an attitude that is critical, bitter,

full of ill-will, to a sour judgment. Nothing disturbs the functioning of the digestion more than that. And it is a vicious circle: the more the digestive function is disturbed, the more unkind you become, critical, dissatisfied with life and things and people. So you can't find any way out. And there is only one cure: to deliberately drop this attitude, to absolutely forbid yourself to have it and to impose upon yourself, by constant self-control, a deliberate attitude of all-comprehending kindness. Just try and you will see that you feel much better.[35]

Egoism*

Several references have been made previously to the inherent disturbances of mental, vital and physical consciousness. However, we become subject to disturbances of mind, vital and body because of an identification with them. From this point of view, these disturbances are related to egoism or the sense of I-ness which becomes attached to these parts of the being. The identification becomes more apparent when one is physically or psychologically unwell, for then one becomes markedly preoccupied with oneself. Hypochondriasis or preoccupation with one's symptoms, associated with any kind of illness, is thus only an accentuation of the constant egoistic state in which we live. As the Mother has pointedly remarked: "Depression is always the sign of an acute egoism. When you feel that it is coming near, tell yourself: 'I am in a state of egoistic illness, I must cure myself of it.' "[36] What has been said here about depression applies to all psychological disturbances — they are different forms of an exacerbated egoistic state.

The egoistic state underlying psychological disturbances

---

* In modern psychology, the ego is conceived of as the self or central core of a person around which all psychological activities revolve. In yoga psychology however, the ego is regarded as the illusory sense of I-ness resulting from an identification of the real self with the body, the emotional nature and the mind. Therefore the term "egoism" which ordinarily means self-centredness or self-pride, does not have that connotation here; it connotes simply a state of identification and its associated sense of I-ness.

is more apparent in certain types of disorders such as mania, paranoia, "inferiority complex", etc. Regarding this last, the Mother plainly points out:

> What gives most the feeling of inferiority, of limitation, smallness, impotence, is always this turning back upon oneself, this shutting oneself up in the bounds of a microscopic ego.[37]

It is interesting to note that the Jungian school of thought attributes mania and depression to abnormal states of the ego, mania being regarded as due to an inflated state, depression due to a deflated state, of the ego. Yoga looks upon mania and depression as related to the rajasic* ego and tamasic† ego respectively. Such a relationship may be gleaned from the following statements in which Sri Aurobindo attributes a number of common symptoms of mania and depression to the rajasic ego and tamasic ego respectively.

> By tamasic ego is meant the ego of weakness, self-depreciation, despondency, unbelief. The rajasic ego is puffed up with pride and self-esteem or stubbornly asserts itself at every step or else wherever it can; the tamasic ego, on the contrary, is always feeling "I am weak, I am miserable, I have no capacity...."[38]

> The tamasic ego is that which accepts and supports despondency, weakness, inertia, self-depreciation, unwillingness to act, unwillingness to know or be open, fatigue, indolence, do-nothingness. Contrary to the rajasic it says, 'I am so weak, so obscure, so miserable, so oppressed and ill-used — there is no hope for me, no success, I am denied everything, am

---

* Characterised by Rajas — the quality of passion and action.

† Characterised by Tamas — the quality of inertia.

‡ These forces have been well known to shamans, medicine-men, occultists, seers and yogis of all times. Sometimes collectively called Satan or the Devil, they are the basis of the belief in possession and the practices of exorcism. Though for centuries relegated by science to the limbo of superstition, these age-old,

unsupported, how can I do this, how can I do that, I have no power for it, no capacity, I am helpless; let me die; let me lie still and moan'.[39]

One quite common psychological disturbance of everyday life related to the ego is over-sensitiveness. "Most sensitiveness", says Sri Aurobindo, "is the result or sign of ego."[40]

Adverse Forces[‡]

Besides internal factors related to the constitutional make-up of the individual, yoga psychology speaks of certain external forces which are involved in some of the psychological disturbances, especially those of a more serious or psychiatric nature. These are spoken of in Integral Yoga as Adverse Forces or Beings of the vital world — the realm of desires and life-energies existing above the material universe. Marked physical or psychological weaknesses create an opening by which a person is influenced, attacked or even possessed by such vital Forces, leading to different types of psychiatric disturbances as explained in the following statements:

> Loss of balance produces disorder in the consciousness and the adverse forces use that loss of balance for attacking and wholly upsetting the system and doing their work. That is why people become hysterical or mad or filled with the desire to die or go away.[41]

> Insanity always indicates possession. The hereditary conditions create a predisposition. It is not possible for a vital Force or Being to invade or take possession unless there are doors open for it to enter. The door may be a vital consent or affinity or

---

universal beliefs and practices have in recent decades been upheld by a few men of science. Perhaps their best known modern exponent in the field of science is the psychiatrist M. Scott Peck, M.D. who in his book, *People of the Lie* (New York: Simon & Schuster, Inc., 1983), has written about "the psychology of evil".

a physical defect in the being.[42]

Insanity is always due to a vital attack, or rather possession although there is often a physical reason as well. Hysteria is due to a pressure from the vital world and there may be momentary possessions also.[43]

Epilepsy is itself a sign of vital attack, even if there is a physical cause for it — the attacking force not being able to disturb the mental and vital (proper) falls on the body and uses some physical cause (latent or growing) for the base of its action. For everything manifested in the physical must have a physical support or means for its expression.[44]

Since, according to Integral Yoga, it is the defects and weaknesses of body, vital and mind in the individual that provide an opening for the action of the vital forces, the *underlying* causes of all disturbances are seen to exist within the individual. Freedom from psychological disturbances can therefore be attained only by developing a state of consciousness other than the physical, vital and mental consciousness which characterizes the "normal" state of the human being. The innermost consciousness — that of the psychic being spoken of earlier — constitutes a state of psychological well-being because it is not only free from disturbances of the physical, the vital, the mental, the subconscient and ego-consciousness, but also immune to the action of the Adverse Forces.

REFERENCES

1. The Mother, *Collected Works of the Mother* (Pondicherry: Sri Aurobindo Ashram, 1972-1987), Vol. 14, p. 292.
2. Sri Aurobindo, *The Synthesis of Yoga*, Sri Aurobindo Birth Centenary Library (hereafter SABCL) (Pondicherry: Sri Aurobindo Ashram, 1970-75), Vol. 20, p. 39.
3. The Mother, *Collected Works of the Mother*, Vol. 12, p. 45.
4. Sri Aurobindo, *Letters on Yoga*, SABCL, Vol. 22, pp. 320-21.

5. Ibid., p. 347.
6. The Mother, *Collected Works of the Mother*, Vol. 9, pp. 303-04.
7. Sri Aurobindo, *Letters on Yoga*, SABCL, Vol. 24, p. 1329.
8. The Mother, *Collected Works of the Mother*, Vol. 4, p. 11.
9. The Mother, *Collected Works of the Mother*, Vol. 6, pp. 258-59.
10. Ibid., p. 319.
11. Ibid., pp. 224-25.
12. Sri Aurobindo, *Letters on Yoga*, SABCL, Vol. 24, p. 1326.
13. The Mother, *Collected Works of the Mother*, Vol. 7, pp. 37-38.
14. The Mother, *Collected Works of the Mother*, Vol. 3, p. 57.
15. The Mother, *Collected Works of the Mother*, Vol. 8, p. 192.
16. M. Friedman and R. H. Rosenman, *Type A Behavior and Your Heart*. New York: Alfred A. Knopf, 1974.
17. The Mother, *Collected Works of the Mother*, Vol. 10, pp. 202-203.
18. The Mother, *Collected Works of the Mother*, Vol. 1, p. 354.
19. The Mother, *Collected Works of the Mother*, Vol. 4, pp. 178-179.
20. Sri Aurobindo, *Letters on Yoga*, SABCL, Vol. 24, pp. 1357-58.
21. The Mother, *Collected Works of the Mother*, Vol. 5, p. 415.
22. Sri Aurobindo, *Letters on Yoga*, SABCL, Vol. 24, p. 1439.
23. Ibid., pp. 1441-42.
24. Ibid., p. 1441.
25. Ibid., p. 1442.
26. Sri Aurobindo, *Letters on Yoga*, SABCL, Vol. 22, p. 348.
27. Sri Aurobindo, *The Life Divine*, SABCL, Vol. 19, pp. 733-34.
28. Sri Aurobindo, *Letters on Yoga*, SABCL, Vol. 22, p. 356.
29. Ibid., p. 357.
30. Ibid., p. 353.
31. Sri Aurobindo, *Letters on Yoga*, SABCL, Vol. 24, p. 1476.
32. The Mother, *Collected Works of the Mother*, Vol. 5, pp. 412-13.
33. The Mother, *Collected Works of the Mother*, Vol. 4, p. 263.
34. Ibid.
35. The Mother, *Collected Works of the Mother*, Vol. 3, p. 292.
36. The Mother, *Collected Works of the Mother*, Vol. 4, p. 10.
37. Ibid., p. 365.
38. Sri Aurobindo, *Letters on Yoga*, SABCL, Vol. 24, p. 1753.
39. Ibid., p. 1381.
40. Ibid., p. 1393.
41. Sri Aurobindo, *Letters on Yoga*, SABCL, Vol. 24, p. 1771.
42. Ibid.
43. Ibid.
44. Ibid.

8 ATTITUDES, MENTAL HEALTH AND YOGA

An attitude is defined as a mental set which predisposes one to *perceive* things in a certain way, to *feel* towards things in a certain way, and to be prone to *react* towards things in a certain way. Thus an attitude influences all the three basic elements of behaviour, namely, thinking, feeling and willing. For example, an attitude of optimism predisposes one to perceive the bright rather than the dark side of things; it tends to make one feel hopeful rather than easily despairing; and it inclines one to continue with one's endeavour rather than to give up effort prematurely. Examples of everyday attitudes which influence behaviour are: optimism or pessimism; courage or timidity; faith or doubt; goodwill or hostility; confidence or diffidence, etc.

The importance of attitudes lies in the fact that they are more potent than external factors in determining success or failure, health or sickness, happiness or unhappiness. As the American psychologist William James (1842-1910) remarked: "The greatest discovery of my generation is that people can change their lives by changing their attitudes of mind." Attitudes are primarily important also because, unlike external factors, over which we generally do not have much control, attitudes lie within us and are therefore susceptible to significant control, given the necessary will and effort.

Most of our attitudes are determined by our predominant feelings. Therefore, how we perceive things and how we are inclined to react towards things depend on how we feel towards things. For the most part, feelings determine attitudes, and attitudes determine behaviour. Thus in most cases, feelings determine behaviour. Psychological disturbances almost always involve harmful feelings, and, consequently, generate attitudes which perpetuate psychological ill-health. Hence the relevance of attitudes for mental health.

From the viewpoint of yoga, attitudes are determined by the predominant state of one's consciousness. What predominates in one's consciousness depends upon the part of one's being with which one is most identified. Most human beings usually identify themselves predominantly with one or another part of the outer being — the body, or the vital (consisting of life energy, impulses, desires, feelings), or the mind. Each of these parts of the being has its own characteristic consciousness and attitudes. The physical consciousness of the body is characterised by inertia, obscurity, mechanical and chaotic activity, repetitiveness, and narrowness or constriction. The vital consciousness is characterized by energism, action and passion. The characteristics of mental consciousness are rationality, objectivity, balance and harmony. The influence of the physical consciousness is to be seen in attitudes which are marked by lethargy, indifference, boredom, doubt, diffidence, depression and pessimism. The vital consciousness is reflected in attitudes which show prejudice or predilection, pride, over-confidence, ambition and excessive optimism. Attitudes stemming from the mental consciousness reflect a rational and objective view of things, and an inclination towards ideals.

All human beings are endowed with physical, vital and mental consciousness, and are therefore influenced by qualities of all the three parts of the outer being in different degrees. But in the majority of people, it is the vital consciousness that is generally predominant, and exercises the strongest influence on their attitudes. From the viewpoint of yoga psychology, the predominance of the vital nature is the chief cause of psychological disturbances. For, the human being at the present stage of evolution is primarily a mental being; therefore to be dominated by the vital being is to act contrary to one's nature as a mental being. So, in order to overcome the force of instincts, impulses, desires and feelings of the vital nature, it is necessary to have recourse to mind and its force of mental will. It is the mind that enables one initially to discriminate between what is beneficial and what is harmful, what is proper and what is improper, what is right and what is wrong. Secondly, the mind, with its force of mental will, can curb, at least to some extent, the instincts and impulses from being expressed in speech or action. Most importantly, mind can formulate and adhere to positive attitudes which one wants to inculcate in oneself. The act of adhering to an attitude and impressing it on one's consciousness by repeating it to oneself — an exercise which is being increasingly used by mental health practitioners — is referred to as affirmation. The practice is akin to auto-suggestion. But auto-suggestion consists in the effort to repeat positive thoughts to oneself while the mind remains relaxed and passive so as to impress these thoughts on what is called the subconscious mind. On the other hand, affirmation involves the mind's active, conscious and deliberate effort to hold on to a positive attitude.

However, from the viewpoint of yoga, it is necessary to go beyond mind if one is truly to succeed in establishing right attitudes. For, though the mind can control the vital nature and prevent its irrational tendencies from dominating one's attitudes, the mind's control is very limited and precarious. Secondly, mental consciousness, being interfused with the physical and the vital consciousness, needs to be freed from their influences before it can express its own rational nature. Most of the time, the lower influences, especially of the vital nature, are so subtle and powerful that the mind is usurped and enslaved by the physical and vital nature, and is even used to defend irrational tendencies by rationalizing them. In order to free itself from domination of the vital nature, mind needs to invoke a force greater than itself. Furthermore, the mind itself has its own inherent disturbances and limitations. To overcome the disturbances and limitations of the mental being, too, a power greater than that of the mind must be tapped, for to try to transform the mind by its own force of mental will and intelligence is, as the well-known simile goes, like trying to cut a knife with its own edge.

Attitudes stemming from a consciousness which is deeper or higher than that of the physical, vital and mental parts of the being are often quite the opposite of the attitudes that prevail in our ordinary consciousness. This may be illustrated from attitudes towards circumstances and towards people around us.

The chief characteristic of the common attitude towards circumstances consists in regarding them as the causes of sorrow or happiness. This attitude is so deeply ingrained in us that most people are not even conscious of it, not to speak of questioning its validity.

Because of such an attitude, people are constantly occupied with trying to change or improve what appear to us to be inimical, unfavourable or less than optimal circumstances. Such an attitude leads to two chief consequences. First, the dependence on circumstances gives them a supremacy and maims the power of the will — the first stage in the development of a neurosis. Secondly, since the attitude that happiness is to be found in favourable circumstances is based on an illusion, people never discover the true inner well-being. As the Mother remarks:

> People think that their condition depends on circumstances. But that is all false. If somebody is a "nervous wreck", he thinks that if circumstances are favourable he will improve. But, actually, even if they are favourable he will remain what he is.... It is not the circumstances that have to be changed: what is required is an inner change.[1]

From the viewpoint of yoga, it is the attitude towards an event or circumstance that determines the kind of effect it has on us. As the Mother categorically states:

> There is a state in which one realises that the effect of things, circumstances, all the movements and actions of life on the consciousness depends almost exclusively upon one's attitude to these things. There is a moment when one becomes sufficiently conscious to realise that things in themselves are truly neither good nor bad: they are this only in relation to us; their effect on us depends absolutely upon the attitude we have towards them. The same thing, identically the same, if we take it as a gift of God, as a divine grace, as the result of the full Harmony, helps us to become more conscious, stronger, more true, while if we take it — exactly the very same circumstance — as a blow from fate, as a bad force wanting to affect us, this constricts us, weighs us down and takes away from us all consciousness and strength and harmony. And the circumstance in itself is *exactly* the same — of this, I should like you all to have the experience, for when you have it, you become master of

yourself. Not only master of yourself but, in what concerns you, master of the circumstances of your life. And this depends exclusively upon the attitude you take.[2]

The right attitude toward circumstances, looked at from the standpoint of yoga, is expressed by Sri Aurobindo in the following letter to a disciple:

> You should not be so dependent on outward things; it is this attitude that makes you give so excessive an importance to circumstances. I do not say that circumstances cannot help or hinder — but they are circumstances, not the fundamental thing which is in ourselves, and their help or their hindrance ought not to be of primary importance. In yoga, as in every great or serious human effort, there is always bound to be an abundance of adverse interventions and unfavourable circumstances which have to be overcome. To give them too great an importance increases their importance and their power to multiply themselves, gives them, as it were, confidence in themselves and the habit of coming. To face them with equanimity — if one cannot manage a cheerful persistence against them of confident and resolute will — diminishes, on the contrary, their importance and effect and in the end, though not at once, gets rid of their persistence and recurrence. It is therefore a principle in yoga to recognise the determining power of what is within us — for that is the deeper truth — to set that right and establish the inward strength as against the power of outward circumstances. The strength is there — even in the weakest; one has to find it, to unveil it and to keep it in front throughout the journey and the battle.[3]

Attitudes towards people around us provide another example of the contrast between ways of looking at them from the ordinary consciousness and from a deeper consciousness. Viewing people from the ordinary consciousness, we tend to admire or idolize some and to criticize or condemn others. From the viewpoint of a deeper consciousness, what we see in others is merely a reflection of what

Attitudes, Mental Health and Yoga 127

we have in ourselves. The good and beautiful qualities which we see and admire in others are potential qualities that lie deeply embedded within us and which we consciously or unconsciously yearn to realize. The dark qualities in others of which we feel critical serve to reflect what we carry in ourselves. As the Mother has well stated it:

> In a general and almost absolute way, anything that shocks you in other people is the very thing you carry in yourself in a more or less veiled, more or less hidden form, though perhaps in a slightly different guise which allows you to delude yourself. And what in yourself seems inoffensive enough, becomes monstrous as soon as you see it in others....
>
> Look upon everything with a benevolent smile. Take all the things which irritate you as a lesson for yourself and your life will be more peaceful and more effective as well, for a great percentage of your energy certainly goes to waste in the irritation you feel when you do not find in others the perfection that you would like to realise in yourself.
>
> You stop short at the perfection that others should realise and you are seldom conscious of the goal you should be pursuing yourself. If you are conscious of it, well then, begin with the work which is given to *you*, that is to say, realise what you have to do and do not concern yourself with what others do, because, after all, it is not your business. And the best way to the true attitude is simply to say, "All those around me, all the circumstances of my life, all the people near me, are a mirror held up to me by the Divine Consciousness to show me the progress I must make. Everything that shocks me in others means a work I have to do in myself."
>
> And perhaps if one carried true perfection in oneself, one would discover it more often in others.[4]

Though yoga calls for rising above the mental consciousness, mind and its will cannot be prematurely abandoned. As Sri Aurobindo remarks: "So long as there is not a constant action of the Force from above or else of a deeper will from within, the mental will is necessary."[5] In dealing with the force of instincts and impulses, what is available to most human beings is the force of mental will. When one undertakes the practice of a spiritual discipline such as yoga, one comes to battle with not only the forces of one's own personal nature, but also with corresponding forces of a universal nature which obstruct or attack the practitioner to subvert the efforts towards rising above the ordinary nature. The importance of using the mind's intelligence and will in dealing with such attacks and obstructions by holding on to the right attitude is pointed out by Sri Aurobindo:

> One sees the negative side only during the attacks, because the first thing the attack or obstruction does is to try to cloud the mind's intelligence. If it cannot do that it is difficult for it to prevail altogether for the time being. For if the mind remains alert and clings to the truth, then the attack can only upheave the vital and, though this may be painful enough, yet the right attitude of the mind acts as a corrective and makes it easier to recover the balance and the true condition of the vital comes back more quickly.[6]

From the evolutionary point of view, the importance of mind lies in the fact that it represents the highest faculty well evolved up to now. Therefore, a certain preparation of the mind is essential for a leap into what is beyond mind. To quote Sri Aurobindo:

> Our evolution has brought the being up out of inconscient Matter into the Ignorance of mind, life and body tempered by an imperfect knowledge and is trying to lead us into the light of the Spirit, to lift us into that light and to bring the light down into us, into body and life as well as mind and heart and to fill with it all that we are. This and its consequences, of which the greatest is the union with the Divine and life in the divine consciousness, is the meaning of the integral transformation. Mind is our present topmost faculty; it is through the thinking mind and the heart with the soul, the psychic being behind them that we have to grow into the Spirit, for what the Force first tries to

bring about is to fix the mind in the right central idea, faith or mental attitude and the right aspiration and poise of the heart and to make these sufficiently strong and firm to last in spite of other things in the mind and heart which are other than or in conflict with them.[7]

What has been stated in the above-quoted passage regarding the action of the Force on the mind for inculcating the right mental attitude is illustrated in the establishment of one of the most important attitudes for mental health as well as for yoga, namely, the attitude of being a detached, uninvolved and non-identified witness of the movements of one's ordinary, surface nature. As Sri Aurobindo states:

> Very often when this witness attitude has not been taken but there is a successful calling in of the Force to act in one, one of the first things the Force does is to establish the witness attitude so as to be able to act with less interference or immixture from the movements of the lower Prakriti.[8]

The practice of affirmation in the field of mental health has been alluded to above. A somewhat similar practice in the field of yoga is the repetition of the *mantra*. Though repeating a *mantra* has a much more profound significance than the practice of affirmation, a feature common to the two practices is that they both serve to inculcate a certain attitude which tends to bring one out of the ordinary, disturbed or constricted state of consciousness. From this limited view-point, a *mantra* may be described as an affirmation that is related to, and which tends to induce, a deeper or higher state of consciousness, impregnated with attitudes of aspiration, courage, hope, trust and faith. The following are examples of mantric affirmations, relevant to a practitioner of yoga:

> Remain fixed in the sunlight of the true consciousness — for only there is happiness and peace. They do not depend upon outside happenings, but on this alone.[9]

> At the very moment when everything seems to go from bad to

worse, it is then that we must make a supreme act of faith and know that the Grace will never fail us.[10]

...in spite of our ignorance and errors and weaknesses and in spite of the attacks of hostile forces and in spite of any immediate appearance of failure the Divine Will is leading us, through every circumstance, towards the final Realisation.[11]

There is a return for all the trials and ordeals of the spiritual life.[12]

Whatever I may be, my soul is a child of the Divine and must reach the Divine sooner or later. I am imperfect, but seek after the perfection of the Divine in me and that not I but the Divine Grace will bring about; if I keep to that the Divine Grace itself will do all.[13]

I want the Divine and nothing else. I want to give myself entirely to him and since my soul wants that, it cannot be but that I shall meet and realise him.[14]

Since I want only the Divine, my success is sure, I have only to walk forward in all confidence and His own Hand will be there secretly leading me to Him by His own way and at His own time.[15]

REFERENCES

1. The Mother, *Collected Works of the Mother* (Pondicherry: Sri Aurobindo Ashram, 1972-1987), Vol. 14, p. 232.
2. The Mother, *Collected Works of the Mother*, Vol. 6, pp. 123-124.
3. Sri Aurobindo, *Letters on Yoga*, Sri Aurobindo Birth Centenary Library (hereafter SABCL) (Pondicherry: Sri Aurobindo Ashram, 1970-75), Vol. 24, p. 1696.
4. The Mother, *Collected Works of the Mother*, Vol. 10, pp. 22-23.
5. Sri Aurobindo, *Letters on Yoga*, SABCL, Vol. 24, p. 1717.
6. Ibid., p. 1753.
7. Ibid., pp. 1624-25.

8. Sri Aurobindo, *Letters on Yoga*, SABCL, Vol. 23, p. 1007.
9. Ibid., SABCL, Vol. 24, p. 1709.
10. The Mother, *Collected Works of the Mother*, Vol. 15, p. 181.
11. Sri Aurobindo, *Letters on Yoga*, SABCL, Vol. 23, p. 579.
12. Ibid., SABCL, Vol. 24, p. 1666.
13. Ibid., p. 1754.
14. Sri Aurobindo, *Letters on Yoga*, SABCL, Vol. 23, p. 587.
15. Ibid., pp. 584-85.

9 MASTERY, MENTAL HEALTH AND YOGA

During the past few decades, the state of mental health has come to be conceived more and more in positive terms, as denoting the presence of certain attributes associated with psychological well-being, rather than the mere absence of a diagnosable disturbance. One such positive view of mental health conceives it as a state of mastery. Perhaps the most prominent among those who have put forth such a view is the psychiatrist, Karl Menninger, who has described human response to life's challenges as consisting of five stages: Panic, Inertia, Striving, Coping, Mastery.* Some of the chief psychological characteristics associated with the five stages are as follows:

Panic: severe anxiety with almost total inability to relax; extreme attachment to things and persons, associated with a strong sense of possessiveness; violent or destructive feelings such as anger, cruelty, jealousy; wanting to possess or destroy others.

Inertia: aimlessness, boredom and depression; living in the past; motivated chiefly by pain-avoidance and the satisfaction of security needs; passivity and indolence; insensitiveness towards the feelings of others.

Striving: struggle to meet one's needs by controlling the environment and persons; motivated chiefly by biological needs; continual stress and tension; not inclined to relax unless compelled; critical of oneself and others; competitive with others.

Coping: motivated by rational goals and interests; more or less successful management of oneself and one's life; a sense of direction, associated with confidence and self-reliance; more relaxed than tense; empathy towards others.

---

* The five stages have been elaborated upon as a measuring scale of mental health by Dr. Wayne Dyer in *The Sky's the Limit*, New York: Pocket Books, 1981.

Mastery: motivated chiefly by ideals, such as Truth, Goodness and Beauty, sense of meaning and purpose in life; poise and centredness; deep sense of security and serenity; great sense of humour; understanding and acceptance of others.

Those familiar with the psychology of yoga would readily detect the correspondence between Panic, Inertia, Striving, Coping, and Mastery on one hand, and the qualities of Tamas, Rajas and Sattwa on the other. Inertia as described above is clearly a state of Tamas, a characteristic attributed in yoga psychology essentially to the physical consciousness. In Sri Aurobindo's words:

> The stigmata of Tamas are blindness and unconsciousness and incapacity and unintelligence, sloth and indolence and inactivity and mechanical routine and the mind's torpor and life's sleep and the soul's slumber....At the heart of this inert impotence is the principle of ignorance and an inability or slothful unwillingness to comprehend, seize and manage the stimulating or assailing contact, the suggestion of environing forces and their urge towards fresh experience.[1]

Both Panic and Striving represent different states of Rajas, the characteristic quality of the vital consciousness. Governed by Rajas, states Sri Aurobindo, a human being is impelled

> ...to strive, to resist, to attempt, to dominate or engross his environment to assert his will, to fight and create and conquer. This is the mode of Rajas, the way of passion and action and the thirst of desire. Struggle and change and new creation, victory and defeat and joy and suffering and hope and disappointment are its children and build the many-coloured house of life in which it takes its pleasure. But its knowledge is an imperfect or a false knowledge and brings with it ignorant effort, error, a constant maladjustment, pain of attachment, disappointed desire, grief of loss and failure.[2]

Coping and Mastery reflect different degrees of the predominance of Sattwa, the quality inherent in mental consciousness. As Sri Aurobindo describes it, Sattwa makes for

> ...clear comprehension, poise and balance... it understands, sympathises; it fathoms and controls and develops Nature's urge and her ways: it has an intelligence that penetrates her processes and her significances and can assimilate and utilise; there is a lucid response that is not overpowered but adjusts, corrects, harmonises, elicits the best in all things. This is the mode of Sattwa, the turn of Nature that is full of light and poise, directed to good, to knowledge, to delight and beauty, to happiness, right understanding, right equilibrium, right order: its temperament is the opulence of a bright clearness of knowledge and lucent warmth of sympathy and closeness. A fineness and enlightenment, a governed energy, an accomplished harmony and poise of the whole being is the consummate achievement of the sattwic nature.[3]

It is interesting to note from the above-stated parallels that Western psychological thought, which began with a highly materialistic view of things based on physiology and biology, representing a polar opposite of the Eastern spiritual viewpoint, is now coming close to the ideas of the East. However, psycho-spiritual concepts like mastery, meditation, disidentification, peace, spontaneity, living in the here and now, etc., which have been recently emerging in Western psychological thought, have a much deeper connotation in the East. This is due to the fact that in the East such concepts are founded on a system of psycho-spiritual thought and discipline, whereas in the West such a foundation is absent. The purpose of this essay is to bring out the deeper implications of the concept of mastery from the viewpoint of the Gita and Sri Aurobindo's yoga.

The Gita regards the ordinary human condition as a state of bondage. Purusha, the Soul, is bound by Prakriti or Nature. As Sri Aurobindo puts it:

> The soul is the witness, upholder, experiencer, but it is master only in theory, in fact it is not-master, *anīśa*, so long as it consents to the Ignorance. For that is a general consent which

implies that the Prakriti gambols about with the Purusha and does pretty well what she likes with him. When he wants to get back his mastery, make the theoretical practical, he needs a lot of tapasya* to do it.[4]

Bondage and limitation are brought about through the operation of the three Gunas — Tamas, Rajas and Sattwa — which are the three essential modes or qualities of Prakriti. Due to Tamas, the mode of inertia and unconsciousness, "man seeks only somehow to survive, to subsist so long as he may, to shelter himself in the fortress of an established routine of thought and action in which he feels himself to a certain extent protected from the battle, able to reject the demand which his higher nature makes upon him, excused from accepting the necessity of farther struggle and the ideal of an increasing effort and mastery."[5] Rajas, the mode of passion, action and struggling emotion leads to "a growth of power and capacity, but it is stumbling, painful, vehement, misled by wrong notions, methods and ideals, impelled to a misuse, corruption and perversion of right notions, methods or ideals, and prone, especially, to a great, often an enormous, exaggeration of the ego."[6] As a result of Sattwa, the mode of poise, knowledge and peace, "there is a more harmonious action, a right dealing with the nature, but right only within the limits of an individual light and a capacity unable to exceed the better forms of this lower mental will and knowledge."[7]

According to the Gita, man's sense of relative freedom and freewill comes from *ahaṁkāra*, the ego, which is itself part of Prakriti and subject to the forces of Prakriti. Thus the will of the ego is not truly a free will, but a will determined by Prakriti, formed in us by the sum of its own past action or Karma. Therefore, the first step towards mastery is freedom of the Purusha from bondage to Prakriti by overcoming the ignorance of identification with Prakriti, and thereby rising above the ego and the Gunas.

In order to rise beyond the action of the Gunas and attain liberation, it is necessary to discover the Purusha and live in its consciousness. Sri Aurobindo explains this as follows:

* Austerity.

> The Purusha or basic consciousness is the true being or at least, in whatever plane it manifests, represents the true being. But in the ordinary nature of man it is covered up by the ego and the ignorant play of the Prakriti and remains veiled behind as the unseen Witness supporting the play of the Ignorance. When it emerges, you feel it as a consciousness behind, calm, central, unidentified with the play which depends on it. It may be covered over, but it is always there. The emergence of the Purusha is the beginning of liberation. But it can also become slowly the Master — slowly because the whole habit of the ego and the play of the lower forces is against that.[8]

One recommendation for the discovery of the true being and its liberation from the surface nature is "the practice of the separation of the Prakriti and the Purusha, the conscious Being standing back detached from all the movements of Nature and observing them as witness and knower and finally as the giver (or refuser) of the sanction and at the highest stage of the development, the Ishwara, the pure will, master of the whole Nature."[9] This practice may appear to be similar to that of disidentification taught in Assagioli's system of Psychosynthesis. However, there is a crucial difference between disidentification as used in psychotherapy and as a spiritual practice. As a psychotherapeutic practice, disidentification generally involves taking one's stand in the mind in trying to distinguish the self from body, feelings and thoughts, and affirming to oneself, "I am not the body, I am not my feelings, I am not my thoughts." Such a practice is helpful in separating oneself to some extent from body, feelings and thoughts, and thereby partially freeing oneself to a small extent from their sway or domination. But as long as the true spiritual being remains veiled by body, feelings and mind, one is inevitably more or less identified with the physical, emotional and mental parts of the surface being. Therefore the partial disidentification one may obtain by exercising one's mental discrimination and mental will breaks down easily, causing one to fall back constantly into the common state of identification. A celebrated passage in the Gita describes the psychological process of this fall into identification in relation to mastery over the senses.

Sri Aurobindo comments on the passage alluded to as follows:

> All intelligent human beings know that they must exercise some control over themselves and nothing is more common than this advice to control the senses; but ordinarily it is only advised imperfectly and practised imperfectly in the most limited and insufficient fashion. Even, however, the sage, the man of clear, wise and discerning soul who really labours to acquire complete self-mastery finds himself hurried and carried away by the senses. That is because the mind naturally lends itself to the senses; it observes the objects of sense with an inner interest, settles upon them and makes them the object of absorbing thought for the intelligence and of strong interest for the will. By that attachment comes, by attachment desire, by desire distress, passion and anger when the desire is not satisfied or is thwarted or opposed, and by passion the soul is obscured, the intelligence and will forget to see and be seated in the calm observing soul; there is a fall from the memory of one's true self, and by that lapse the intelligent will is also obscured, destroyed even. For, for the time being, it no longer exists to our memory of ourselves, it disappears in a cloud of passion; we become passion, wrath, grief and cease to be self and intelligence and will.[10]

As a spiritual practice, disidentification involves not merely the negative process of distinguishing body, feelings and mind as the not-self, but rather, a positive identification with the true spiritual being. Such an identification can be achieved, not by mere mental exercise, but by an all-absorbing concentration and an all-consuming aspiration for transcendence of the mind and dissolution of the ego. Herein lies a fundamental difference between yoga and psychotherapeutic approaches in general. The latter utilise the positive aspects of mind and ego for overcoming psychological disturbances or for promoting psychological growth. From the viewpoint of yoga, however, identification with mind and ego implies ignorance about one's true being. Such ignorance inevitably entails limitation, bondage and suffering. The higher aspects of mind and feeling can indeed bring some amelioration of the suffering, as they also can lead to a relative mastery. But true well-being and real mastery come only from the Self. These teachings of the Gita, variously expressed thus far, are succinctly recapitulated in the following passage:

> When we can live in the higher Self... we become superior to the method of the lower workings of Prakriti. We are no longer enslaved to Nature and her Gunas, but, one with the Ishwara, the master of our nature, we are able to use her without subjection to the chain of Karma, for the purposes of the Divine Will in us; for that is what the Greater Self in us is, he is the Lord of her works and unaffected by the troubled stress of her reactions. The soul ignorant in Nature, on the contrary, is enslaved by that ignorance to her modes, because it is identified there, not felicitously with its true self, not with the Divine who is seated above her, but stupidly and unhappily with the ego-mind which is a subordinate factor in her operations in spite of the exaggerated figure it makes, a mere mental knot and point of reference for the play of the natural workings. To break this knot, no longer to make the ego the centre and beneficiary of our works, but to derive all from and refer all to the divine Supersoul is the way to become superior to all the restless trouble of Nature's modes. For it is to live in the supreme consciousness, of which the ego-mind is a degradation, and to act in an equal and unified Will and Force and not in the unequal play of the Gunas which is a broken seeking and striving, a disturbance, an inferior Maya.[11]

Bondage and mastery have thus far been explained from the viewpoint of the Gita in terms of Purusha, Prakriti, Gunas and Ishwara. Sri Aurobindo introduces another cardinal concept pertaining to the psychology of mastery — that of the psychic being. The psychic being is Chaitya Purusha, the Purusha in the heart, which constitutes the inmost being, as distinguished from the inner being which consists of Annamaya Purusha (the Purusha in the physical), Pranamaya Purusha (the Purusha in the vital) and Manomaya

Purusha (the Purusha in the mental). The outer, the inner and the inmost parts of the being are spoken of in the following extract which alludes to mastery:

> There are, we might say, two beings in us, one on the surface, our ordinary exterior mind, life, body consciousness, another behind the veil, an inner mind, an inner life, an inner physical consciousness constituting another or inner self. This inner self once awake opens in its turn to our true real eternal self. It opens inwardly to the soul, called in the language of this yoga the psychic being which supports our successive births and at each birth assumes a new mind, life and body. It opens above to the Self or Spirit which is unborn and by conscious recovery of it we transcend the changing personality and achieve freedom and full mastery over our nature.[12]

According to Sri Aurobindo's Yoga, the psychic being is a portion of the Divine and is thus the Ishwara of our individual nature. Therefore the key to mastery over one's outer being and life lies in discovering the psychic and bringing it to the front. This is expressed in the following statements:

> The outer being, left to itself, is not very responsible; it is most often the plaything of the forces of Nature. But the inner or higher being, the deeper consciousness, is the master and builder of our destiny. That is why it is so important to discover this sovereign consciousness and unite with it in order to put an end to all the incoherencies of life and all the conflicts of Nature.[13]

> To be aware of one's central consciousness and to know the action of the forces is the first definite step towards self-mastery.[14]

> ...the first step is the identification, and then, once you can keep this identification, the psychic governs the rest of the nature and life. It becomes the master of existence. So this is

what we mean by the psychic coming in front. It is that which governs, directs, even organises the life, organises the consciousness, the different parts of the being.[15]

The most important thing for an individual is to unify himself around his divine centre; in that way he becomes a true individual, master of himself and his destiny. Otherwise, he is a plaything of forces that toss him about like a piece of cork on a river. He goes where he does not want to go, he is made to do things he does not want to do, and finally, he loses himself in a hole without having any strength to recover. But if you are consciously organised, unified around the divine centre, ruled and directed by it, you are master of your destiny.[16]

In ordinary life, human beings try to control undesirable feelings, thoughts and actions with the help of mental intelligence and mental will. However, too often the mind is unable to discern what is undesirable, and even when it can so discern, the mental will is often too weak to overcome the wrong movement. The psychic, on the other hand, has an immediate perception of what is right and wrong, and has an inherent power to reject automatically what is wrong. That is why the practice of yoga involves a progressive replacement of the mental control by psychic and spiritual self-mastery. As Sri Aurobindo states:

In sadhana* the mental or moral control has to be replaced by the spiritual mastery — for that mental control is only partial and it controls but does not liberate; it is only the psychic and spiritual that can do that. This is the main difference in this respect between the ordinary and the spiritual life.[17]

Your difficulty in getting rid of the aboriginal in your nature will remain so long as you try to change your vital part by the sole or main strength of your mind and mental will, calling in at most an indefinite and impersonal divine power to aid you....

---

* The practice of yoga.

If you want a true mastery and transformation of the vital movements, it can be done only on condition you allow your psychic being, the soul in you, to awake fully, to establish its rule and opening all to the permanent touch of the Divine Shakti*....[18]

It should be evident from what has been stated above that the concept of mastery in yoga is much deeper than what it connotes in the West. It may be said that in the West, mastery, like other terms used to delineate the positive state of mental health, describes a quality of being which in the language of the Gita would be called sattwic. Most human beings fall short of such an ideal state because they are governed primarily by Tamas and Rajas. However, from the viewpoint of yoga, the mastery conferred by Sattwa is only a relative one, since Sattwa too is a quality of Prakriti, the outer nature, which in our present state of Ignorance binds the Purusha, the true inner being. As Sri Aurobindo states:

> ...richness of life, even a sattwic harmony of mind and nature does not constitute spiritual perfection.... Sattwa itself does not give the highest or the integral perfection; Sattwa is always a quality of the limited nature; sattwic knowledge is the light of a limited mentality, sattwic will is the government of a limited intelligent force. Moreover, Sattwa cannot act by itself in Nature, but has to rely for all action on the aid of Rajas, so that even sattwic action is always liable to the imperfections of Rajas; egoism, perplexity, inconsistency, a one-sided turn, a limited and exaggerated will, exaggerating itself in the intensity of its limitations, pursue the mind and action even of the saint, philosopher and sage. There is a sattwic as well a rajasic or tamasic egoism, at the highest an egoism of knowledge or virtue; but the mind's egoism of whatever type is incompatible with liberation. All the three gunas have to be transcended. Sattwa may bring us near to the Light, but its limited clarity falls away from us when we enter into the luminous body of the divine Nature.[19]

* Power.

Thus, according to yoga, true mastery can be attained only by becoming *trigunātīta*, above and beyond the three Gunas, by disidentifying from Prakriti, and attaining "the true character of the Purusha, free, master, knower, and enjoyer."[20] For mastery lies in "the power of the internal consciousness — above as Atman, below as Purusha first witness and then master of the nature."[21]

As implied in the last quotation, the state of mastery is preceded by the witness state of liberation in which one becomes a detached, unidentified observer, unaffected by whatever takes place in the outer being and external environment. This is one of the methods taught in yoga for gaining control over the mind. Thus, in a letter to a disciple, Sri Aurobindo advises:

> Detach yourself from it [the habitual movement of thoughts] — make your mind external to it, something that you can observe as you observe things occurring in the street. So long as you do not do that it is difficult to be the mind's master.[22]

But detachment must culminate in a still higher state before one can be said to have attained mastery. The distinction between detachment and mastery is explained by Sri Aurobindo thus:

> Detachment is the beginning of mastery, but for complete mastery there should be no reactions at all. When there is something within undisturbed by the reactions that means the inner being is free and master of itself, but it is not yet master of the whole nature. When it is master, it allows no wrong reactions — if any come they are at once repelled and shaken off, and finally none come at all.[23]

In the language of the Gita, the Purusha has a higher status than even that of the free and passive witness, *sāksi*. By rising to that higher status one becomes Swarat, self-ruler, the Ishwara, Lord and Master. "When that is done, the Purusha is no longer only a witness, but also the master of his prakriti, *īśvara*."[24]

REFERENCES

1. Sri Aurobindo, *The Synthesis of Yoga*, Sri Aurobindo Birth Centenary Library (hereafter SABCL) (Pondicherry: Sri Aurobindo Ashram, 1970-75), Vol. 20, p. 221.
2. Ibid., pp. 221-22.
3. Ibid., p. 222.
4. Sri Aurobindo, *Letters on Yoga*, SABCL, Vol. 24, p. 1111.
5. Sri Aurobindo, *Essays on the Gita*, SABCL, Vol. 13, p. 49.
6. Ibid., p. 358.
7. Ibid.
8. Sri Aurobindo, *Letters on Yoga*, SABCL, Vol. 23, p. 1006.
9. Ibid., p. 673.
10. Sri Aurobindo, *Essays on the Gita*, SABCL, Vol. 13, pp. 93-94.
11. Ibid., p. 202.
12. Sri Aurobindo, *Letters on Yoga*, SABCL, Vol. 23, pp. 1020-21.
13. The Mother, *Collected Works of the Mother* (Pondicherry: Sri Aurobindo Ashram, 1972-1987), Vol. 14, p. 357.
14. Sri Aurobindo, *Letters on Yoga*, SABCL, Vol. 23, p. 1011.
15. The Mother, *Collected Works of the Mother*, Vol. 6, p. 334.
16. The Mother, *Collected Works of the Mother*, Vol. 5, p. 139.
17. Sri Aurobindo, *Letters on Yoga*, SABCL, Vol. 24, p. 1298.
18. Ibid., pp. 1532-33.
19. Sri Aurobindo, *The Synthesis of Yoga*, SABCL, Vol. 21, p. 660.
20. Sri Aurobindo, *The Synthesis of Yoga*, SABCL, Vol. 20, p. 92.
21. Sri Aurobindo, *Letters on Yoga*, SABCL, Vol. 24, p. 1441.
22. Ibid., pp. 1268-69.
23. Sri Aurobindo, *Letters on Yoga*, SABCL, Vol. 23, p. 1012.
24. Sri Aurobindo, *The Synthesis of Yoga*, SABCL, Vol. 21, p. 739.

10 THE HEALING POWER OF PEACE

> *For everything — to live the spiritual life, heal sickness — for everything, one must be calm.*[1]
>
> THE MOTHER

There has been a growing recognition of the role of stress in producing physical illness as well as psychiatric disturbances. According to conservative estimates, about fifty to seventy per cent of all physical illnesses and a substantial percentage of psychiatric disturbances are related to stress. As a result, a number of therapeutic approaches for stress reduction and for the treatment of stress-related disorders have come into vogue during the past few decades. Some of the chief techniques used today include Progressive Relaxation, Autogenic Training, Relaxation Response, Biofeedback, the use of visual imagery, and breathing. The common feature of these and other similar methods is that they all serve to restore the homeostatic balance disrupted by stress.

Walter B. Cannon, who pioneered the study of the physiological reaction to stress, traced the basis of the stress reaction to an adaptive response made by the autonomic nervous system when an organism is faced with a life-threatening situation. Faster breathing, quicker pumping of the blood by the heart, an easier coagulation of the blood and other bodily changes brought about by the release of adrenalin have come to be seen as adaptive functions in the face of a life-threatening danger, because such emergency reactions give an animal organism the extra strength needed to fight the danger or run away from it, and to reduce the chances of bleeding to death in the case of injury. Therefore, Cannon called it a "fight or flight" reaction. This oft-quoted phrase contains a hint regarding the relevance of peace in healing stress-related disorders, for peace is the state antithetical to that produced by a "fight or flight" reaction.

The physiological reaction opposite to that of "fight or flight" was not named until relatively recently when Herbert Benson coined the phrase "relaxation response" to describe a state in which breathing is slow and deep, the heart-rate is slowed down, the muscles are relaxed and there is a feeling of relaxation. In the writer's opinion, this state of relaxation is a diminutive physiological form of the spiritual state of peace.

Peace, like relaxation, is generally understood as the absence of restlessness or tension rather than as a positive state with its own content. This seems to be due to the fact that our experience of peace is rarely deep enough to make us aware of its positive nature. In truth, however, to regard peace merely as the absence of disturbance is similar to looking upon joy as the absence of suffering. Peace, like joy, has a positive content of its own, and is a powerful force that works for harmony and healing. As the Mother says:

> Quietude is a very positive state; there is a positive peace which is not the opposite of conflict — an active peace, contagious, powerful, which controls and calms, which puts everything in order, organises.... True quietude is a very great force, a very great strength.[2]

Quietude, calm and peace are the one panacea that time and again have been prescribed in yoga for all maladies, physical and psychological. Here are some statements to this effect:

> Peace and stillness are the great remedy for disease. When we can bring peace in our cells, we are cured.[3]

> Catch hold of a peace deep within and push it into the cells of the body. With the peace will come back the health.[4]

> The imperative condition for cure is calm and quietness. Any agitation, any nervousness prolongs the illness.[5]

The rationale for the efficacy of peace in healing lies in the fact that illness is essentially a state of disequilibrium, and peace is a sovereign remedy for establishing equilibrium. As the Mother states:

> In reality illness is only a disequilibrium; if then you are able

to establish another equilibrium, this disequilibrium disappears. An illness is simply, always, in every case, even when the doctors say that there are microbes — in every case, a disequilibrium in the being: a disequilibrium among the various functions, a disequilibrium among the forces.[6]

The exact way in which disequilibrium brings in illness, and how peace can act as a healing force is explained in the following passage:

> The vital body surrounds the physical body with a kind of envelope which has almost the same density as the vibrations of heat observable when the day is very hot. And it is this which is the intermediary between the subtle body and the most material vital body. It is this which protects the body from all contagion, fatigue, exhaustion and even from accidents. Therefore if this envelope is wholly intact, it protects you from everything, but a little too strong an emotion, a little fatigue, some dissatisfaction or any shock whatsoever is sufficient to scratch it as it were and the slightest scratch allows any kind of intrusion. Medical science also now recognises that if you are in perfect vital equilibrium, you do not catch illness or in any case you have a kind of immunity from contagion. If you have this equilibrium, this inner harmony which keeps the envelope intact, it protects you from everything. There are people who lead quite an ordinary life, who know how to sleep as one should, eat as one should, and their nervous envelope is so intact that they pass through all dangers as though unconcerned. It is a capacity one can cultivate in oneself. If one becomes aware of the weak spot in one's envelope, a few minutes' concentration, a call to the force,* an inner peace is sufficient for it to be all right, get cured, and for the untoward thing to vanish.[7]

The above passage further implies that peace is a power for not only healing but also for prevention. For, the most important factor

---

* The Divine Force.

in prevention is one's power of resistance to disease. This power to ward off illness depends not so much on physical strength as on inner strength which, the Mother states, is always associated with calm and peace.

> ...all those who are really strong, powerful, are always very calm. It is only the weak who are agitated; as soon as one becomes truly strong, one is peaceful, calm, quiet.... This true quietude is always a sign of force. Calmness belongs to the strong.[8]

The relevance of such strength in preventing illness is indicated in the following statement:

> Establish a greater peace and quietness in your body, that will give you the strength to resist attacks of illness.[9]

In other words, it is an inner weakness, associated with agitation and restlessness, that leads to a lowered resistance and makes one vulnerable to disease. In this regard, the Mother makes a striking observation: "...the most important of all causes for bodily illness is that the body begins to get restless."[10] Therefore, the first measure recommended for curing oneself of a bodily illness is bringing peace to the part that is ailing. She states:

> ...we said that this disharmony creates a kind of tremor and a lack of peace in the physical being, in the body. It is a kind of fever. Even if it is not a fever in general, there is a localised fever; there are people who get restless. So the first thing to do is to quieten oneself, bring peace, calm, relaxation, with a total confidence, in this little corner (not necessarily in the whole body).[11]

The last statement, like several others quoted earlier, contains an important implication regarding the nature of peace. Generally, peace is thought of as something which is psychological, that is, pertaining to a state of the mind or feelings. However, the integral peace that the Mother speaks about pertains also to the body. She therefore sometimes uses the term "immobility" when referring to peace in the body. The following passage describes how nerve pain can be overcome by immobility:

> ...if one can do two things: either bring into oneself — for all nervous suffering, for example — bring into oneself a kind of immobility, as total as possible, at the place of pain, this has the effect of an anaesthetic. If one succeeds in bringing an inner immobility, an immobility of the inner vibration, at the spot where one is suffering, it has exactly the same effect as an anaesthetic. It cuts off the contact between the place of pain and the brain, and once you have cut the contact, if you keep this state long enough, the pain will disappear... And then, if you can add to that a kind of inner peace and a trust that the pain will go away, well, I tell you that it will go.[12]

Such overcoming of pain by means of immobility, unlike the suppressive measures of pain-killing drugs, is not only free from harmful side-effects associated with drugs, but can have also a deeper action that is more than a mere temporary palliative. The Mother states that an inner mastery over pain can also lead to a permanent cure of the underlying condition which produces the pain. She says:

> And there are a number of illnesses or states of physical imbalance which can be cured simply by removing the effect, that is, by stopping the suffering. Usually it comes back because the cause is still there. If the cause of the illness is found and one acts directly on its cause, then one can be cured radically. But if one is not able to do that, one can make use of this influence, of this control over pain in order — by cutting off the pain or eliminating it or mastering it in oneself — to work on the illness.[13]

There has been some clinical research which seems to corroborate the therapeutic efficacy of immobility. K. K. Datey and his colleagues have demonstrated that the yogic posture Shavasana significantly reduces blood pressure in hypertensive patients.[14] Similar results have been reported by the cardiologist Chandra H. Patel who employed Shavasana in conjunction with biofeedback.[15]

The rationale for the therapeutic effects of Shavasana has not been adequately explained. The muscular relaxation involved in the posture seems to be only part of the explanation. This writer is inclined to believe that a good deal of the therapeutic value of the "corpse posture" lies in the state of immobility produced by making the body as still as a corpse.

It has been stated earlier that we are not generally aware of the positive nature of peace because our experience of peace is rarely deep enough. But another probable reason is that we are used to thinking of a positive force as dynamic, that is, as something which is expressed in action or movement rather than in stillness or immobility. In other words, it is difficult for us to conceive of power as static. As the Mother observes:

> ...a human being becomes aware of power only when it is dynamic; a human being doesn't consider it a power except when it acts; if it doesn't act he does not even notice it, he does not realise the tremendous force which is behind this inaction — at times, even frequently, a force more formidable than the power which acts.[16]

The difference between static and dynamic power is explained in the following passage:

> ...there is the same difference between static power and dynamic power as between a game of defence and a game of attack.... Static power is something which can withstand everything, nothing can act upon it, nothing can touch it, nothing can shake it — it is immobile, but it is invincible. Dynamic power is something in action, which at times goes forth and may at times receive blows. That is to say, if you want your dynamic power to be always victorious, it must be supported by a considerable static power, an unshakable base.[17]

Many of the physical and psychological maladies of our times may be conceived of as stemming from an excessive dynamism without a base of static power in the form of an inner poise. This seems to be supported by the findings of Friedman and Rosenman, two cardiologists who have concluded that the classic American life-style — the hard-driving pursuit of success — is the key to America's soaring rate of coronary disease.[18] According to these two researchers, traits which constitute what they call Type A behaviour are a major factor in heart attacks — more important than obesity, high blood pressure and smoking. The two chief characteristics of Type A behaviour, according to Friedman and Rosenman, are "hurry sickness" and an inordinate drive toward achievement, usually associated with competition. Persons with Type A behaviour pattern, say the two authors, are "involved in a *chronic, incessant* struggle to achieve more and more in less and less time...."[19]

In these findings may be discerned a striking closeness to the following observations made by the Mother about ten years prior to the publication of the book by Friedman and Rosenman:

> ...they [men] are always wanting — quick, quick, quick — to rush from one thing to another, to do one thing quickly and move on to the next one.... They are always wanting: forward, forward, forward....
>
> And I have observed this in the cells of the body; they always seem to be in a hurry to do what they have to do, lest they have no time to do it.... Muddled people...have this to a high degree, this kind of haste — quick, quick, quick.... You go hurtling through life... to go where?... You end with a crash![20]

The remedy suggested by the Mother for this "hurry sickness" is the same as always. She says:

> ...to live to the utmost of one's capacities at every minute, without planning or wanting, waiting or preparing for the next....
>
> All those who have tried to be wise have always said it — the Chinese preached it, the Indians preached it — to live in the awareness of Eternity. In Europe also they said that one should contemplate the sky and the stars and identify oneself

with their infinitude — all things that widen you and give you peace.[21]

The Mother does not advocate a flight from action in order to find peace. Her gospel is one of action and dynamism. She speaks, however, of the need for finding "rest in action":

Become as vast as the world and you will always be at rest. In the thick of action, in the very midst of the battle, the effort, you will know the repose of infinity and eternity.[22]

How to establish peace within oneself? Here is how the Mother answered the question on one occasion in talking to the children in the Ashram:

First of all, you must want it.
And then you must try and must persevere, continue trying. What I have just told you is a very good means. Yet there are others also. You sit quietly, to begin with; and then, instead of thinking of fifty things, you begin saying to yourself, "Peace, peace, peace, peace, peace, calm, peace!" You imagine peace and calm. You aspire, ask that it may come: "Peace, peace, calm." And then, when something comes and touches you and acts, say quietly, like this, "Peace, peace, peace." Do not look at the thoughts, do not listen to the thoughts, you understand. You must not pay attention to everything that comes. You know, when someone bothers you a great deal and you want to get rid of him, you don't listen to him, do you? Good! You turn your head away (*gesture*) and think of something else. Well, you must do that: when thoughts come, you must not look at them, must not listen to them, must not pay any attention at all, you must behave as though they did not exist, you see! And then, repeat all the time like a kind of — how shall I put it? — as an idiot does, who repeats the same thing always. Well, you must do the same thing; you must repeat, "Peace, peace, peace." So you try this for a few minutes and then do what you have to do; and then, another time, you begin again; sit down again and

then try. Do this on getting up in the morning, do this in the evening when going to bed... if you want to digest your food properly, you can do this for a few minutes before eating. You can't imagine how much this helps your digestion!... and there comes a time when you no longer need to sit down, and no matter what you are doing, no matter what you are saying, it is always "Peace, peace, peace." Everything remains here, like this, it does not enter (*gesture in front of the forehead*), it remains like this. And then one is always in a perfect peace... after some years.

But at the beginning, a very small beginning, two or three minutes, it is very simple. For something complicated you must make an effort, and when one makes an effort, one is not quiet. It is difficult to make an effort while remaining quiet. Very simple, very simple, you must be very simple in these things. It is as though you were learning how to call a friend: by dint of being called he comes. Well, make peace and calm your friends and call them: "Come, peace, peace, peace, peace, come!"[23]

To those who are engaged in the practice of Sadhana, illness may sometimes come because of lack of enough receptivity to the spiritual forces which one calls down by one's aspiration. The method of relieving such a disturbance is essentially the same, and consists in relaxing the part of the being (physical, vital, or mental), where there is resistance to the higher forces, by using one's will, or by widening the consciousness or simply by calling the peace. The Mother speaks about this in the following passage:

> The method is almost the same for all parts of the being. To begin with, the first condition: to remain as quiet as possible. You may notice that in the different parts of your being, when something comes and you do not receive it, this produces a shrinking — there is something which hardens in the vital, the mind or the body. There is a stiffening and this hurts, one feels a mental, vital or physical pain. So, the first thing is to put one's will and relax this shrinking, as one does a twitching nerve or a

The Healing Power of Peace

cramped muscle; you must learn how to relax, be able to relieve this tension in whatever part of the being it may be.

The method of relaxing the contraction may be different in the mind, the vital or the body, but logically it is the same thing. Once you have relaxed the tension, you see first if the disagreeable effect ceases, which would prove that it was a small momentary resistance, but if the pain continues and if it is indeed necessary to increase the receptivity in order to be able to receive what is helpful, what should be received, you must, after having relaxed this contraction, begin trying to widen yourself — you feel you are widening yourself. There are many methods. Some find it very useful to imagine they are floating on water with a plank under their back. Then they widen themselves, widen, until they become the vast liquid mass. Others make an effort to identify themselves with the sky and the stars, so they widen, widen themselves, identifying themselves more and more with the sky. Others again don't need these pictures; they can become conscious of their consciousness, enlarge their consciousness more and more until it becomes unlimited. One can enlarge it till it becomes vast as the earth and even the universe. When one does that one becomes really receptive.... One can act through thought, by calling the peace, tranquillity (the feeling of peace takes away much of the difficulty) like this: "Peace, peace, peace... tranquillity... calm." Many discomforts, even physical, like all these contractions of the solar plexus, which are so unpleasant and give you at times nausea, the sensation of being suffocated, of not being able to breathe again, can disappear thus. It is the nervous centre which is affected, it gets affected very easily. As soon as there is something which affects the solar plexus, you must say, "Calm... calm... calm", become more and more calm until the tension is destroyed.[24]

The Mother's prescription of peace as a sovereign remedy for preventing as well as healing physical and psychological disorders is based on the occult knowledge of vibrations. In a passage previously quoted, the Mother alludes to vibrations of disorder as producing a "tremor...in the body" and causing "a kind of fever".[25] In another previously quoted passage,[26] an allusion to vibrations was made in speaking about having "observed this in the cells of the body...in a hurry to do what they have to do".

We are not aware of these vibrations, "but the body trembles, and one doesn't know it, because it is in the cells of the body that the trembling goes on. It trembles with a terrible anxiety and this is what attracts the illness."[27]

All illnesses, according to the Mother, are characterized by such vibrations of disorder. She describes the external source of an illness as "a kind of vibration made up of a mental suggestion, a vital force of disorder and certain physical elements which are the materialisation of the mental suggestion and the vital vibration. And these physical elements can be what we have agreed to call germs, microbes, this and that and many other things."[28]

"If you could see that kind of dance, the dance of vibrations which is there around you all the time, you would see, would understand well what I mean."[29]

According to the Mother, even accidents are the aftermath of harmful vibrations. She says:

> ...in a game, when you play, it is like this (*gesture*), and then it is like the vibrations of a point, it goes on increasing, increasing and increasing until suddenly, crash!...an accident. And it is a collective atmosphere like that; we come and see it, you are in the midst of a game — basketball or football or any other — we feel it, see it, it produces a kind of smoke around you (those vapours of heat which come at times, something like that), and then it takes on a vibration like that, like that, more and more, more and more, more and more until suddenly the equilibrium is broken: someone breaks his leg, falls down, is hit on the mouth by a ball, etc. And one can foretell beforehand that this is going to happen when it is like that. But nobody is aware of it.[30]

As stated earlier, susceptibility to noxious vibrations from outside is due to negative vibrations within oneself. Therefore the only way to protect oneself from succumbing to an illness is to establish harmony within oneself. And in order to do this one needs first to become aware of vibrations of disharmony within oneself. Often people are not aware of a disorder until it manifests itself in the form of gross physical symptoms such as headache, fever, pain, swelling, etc. When one is a little more conscious and sensitive, one feels an inner malaise before one develops gross physical symptoms. But if one is to use the power of peace for preventing an attack of illness, one needs to cultivate one's consciousness a step further and become aware of the *constant* play of vibrations, both internal and external. If one can cultivate such awareness and can *constantly* establish a peaceful vibration within oneself, one renders oneself immune to all attacks.

Such a rationale regarding the cause and prevention — as well as the healing — of a disorder in terms of vibrations is summed up in the Mother's following statements:

> ...there is always a way of isolating oneself by an atmosphere of protection, if one knows how to have an extremely quiet vibration, so quiet that it makes almost a kind of wall around you. — But all the time, all the time one is vibrating in response to vibrations which come from outside. If you become aware of this all the time there is something which does this (*gesture*),... which responds to all the vibrations coming from outside. You are never in an absolutely quiet atmosphere which emanates from you, that is, which comes from inside outward (not something which comes from outside within), something which is like an envelope around you, very quiet, like this — and you can go anywhere at all and these vibrations which come from outside do not begin to do this (*gesture*) around your atmosphere.[31]

> ...and it is only when you have this conscious, extremely calm atmosphere, and as I say, when it comes from within (it is not something that comes from outside), it is only when it's like this that you can go with impunity into life, that is, among others and in all the circumstances of every minute....[32]

REFERENCES

1. The Mother, *Collected Works of the Mother* (Pondicherry: Sri Aurobindo Ashram, 1972-1987), Vol. 4, p. 271.
2. The Mother, *Collected Works of the Mother*, Vol. 8, p. 330.
3. The Mother, *Collected Works of the Mother*, Vol. 15, p. 163.
4. Ibid.
5. Ibid.
6. The Mother, *Collected Works of the Mother*, Vol. 5, p. 122.
7. The Mother, *Collected Works of the Mother*, Vol. 4, p. 63.
8. The Mother, *Collected Works of the Mother*, Vol. 8, p. 330.
9. The Mother, *Collected Works of the Mother*, Vol. 15, p. 161.
10. The Mother, *Collected Works of the Mother*, Vol. 5, p. 176.
11. Ibid., p. 186.
12. The Mother, *Collected Works of the Mother*, Vol. 6, pp. 407-8.
13. Ibid., p. 406.
14. K. K. Datey, S. M. Deshmukh, D. P. Dalvi and S. L. Vinekar, "Shavasan, a yogic exercise in the management of hypertension". *Angiology*, 20 (1969), pp. 325-33.
15. C. H. Patel, "Yoga and biofeedback in the management of hypertension". *Lancet* (Nov. 10, 1973).
16. The Mother, *Collected Works of the Mother*, Vol. 4, p. 368.
17. Ibid.
18. M. Friedman and R. H. Rosenman, *Type A Behavior and Your Heart*. New York: Alfred A. Knopf, 1974.
19. Ibid., p. 84.
20. The Mother, *Collected Works of the Mother*, Vol. 10, pp. 202-3.
21. Ibid., p. 203.
22. The Mother, *Collected Works of the Mother*, Vol. 9, p. 65.
23. The Mother, *Collected Works of the Mother*, Vol. 6, pp. 313-14.
24. The Mother, *Collected Works of the Mother*, Vol. 4, pp. 265-66.
25. Vide reference 11.
26. Vide reference 20.
27. The Mother, *Collected Works of the Mother*, Vol. 7, p. 145.
28. Ibid., p. 146.
29. Ibid., p. 147.
30. Ibid.
31. Ibid., pp. 146-47.
32. Ibid., p. 147.

INDEX

Abulia   105
Accidents   146, 154
Adler, Alfred   11, 29, 47
Adverse (vital) Forces   118-20
   possession by   118-19fn
Affirmation   124, 129-30
Anger   79, 80, 107
Anxiety (worry)   78-79, 100-01, 107
Archetype(s)   26-27, 47, 85
Assagioli, Roberto   50, 59, 75, 136
Attitude(s)   122-31
   and behaviour   122
   and circumustances   124-26
   witness   129
Auto-suggestion   124
Awareness
   and consciousness   53-55
   and identification   62

Behaviour
   and archetypes   47
   and attitudes   122
   and insight   55
   motivating forces in,   11-12
Behaviourism   13-15
   and psychoanalysis   14
Being
   fullness of   56
   individual and universal   54
   inner   37, 38-39, 139
   parts of   29, 51, 74-75
   planes of   98
   surface (outer)   31-32, 38-39
Benson, Herbert   144
Bergson   11
Berne, Eric   48, 49
Bioenergetics   82
Breuer, Joseph   25
Buddha   106

Cannon, Walter B.   144

Capra, Fritjof   46
Christine Sister   89
Consciousness
   and attitudes   122-23
   and awareness   53, 54-55
   concept of   52-53
   cosmic   52
   and ego   19, 20, 52
   essence of existence   53
   evolution of   29-30
   mental, and attitudes   117
   mental, rising above   121
   and mind   19, 32
   objectivising consciousness and anxiety   100
   physical   98-99, 111-12, 113
      and attitudes   123
   science of   17-18, 21
   and self   54-55
   spectrum of   19, 20, 52
   vital, and attitudes   123
   widening   65

Datey, K.K.   148
Defence mechanisms   77-78, 101-103
Depth psychology   5, 13, 52
Depression   79, 80, 107, 108fn, 117-18
Desire(s)   106-07, 110
Detachment   142; *cf.* Witness attitude
Disidentification   136-37, 142
Doubt   104-05
Dreams   34, 35, 39
Drug addiction   114
Dyer, Dr. Wayne   132fn

Ego (egoism)   19-20, 26, 46, 60, 117-18, 135, 136, 137, 144
   and being   18
   and consciousness   19, 20, 52

and disturbances 117-18
and freewill 135-36
and identification 65, 66
and over-sensitiveness 118
Ellis, Albert 49-50
Epilepsy 119
Evolution 29-30

Fear 107
Freud, Sigmund 5, 7, 25-26, 47, 48, 49, 52, 79
  and Jung 11, 27-29
  on repetition compulsion 7, 35-36, 113
  on repression 6, 25-26
  and Sri Aurobindo 11-13, 35-36
  on the unconscious 5, 25, 26, 42
Friedman, M. 79, 108, 150

Gestalt Therapy 48, 82
Gita, the 86, 92, 134, 135, 136, 138, 141, 142
Gunas 135, 138, 142

Habit 112, 114
Hartmann, E. Von 24
Holmes, T.H. 109
Humanistic Psychology 16-17
Hysteria 119

Identification 58-69, 137, 138, 139
  and awareness 62
  conscious, methods of 66-67
  for curing nervous diseases 66
  and the ego 65, 66
  and knowledge 61-62, 62-63, 64, 66, 67-68
  two types of 61-66
Illness(es) 145-46, 147
  chronic 114
  curing oneself 147
  and stress 144
  and vibrations of disorder 153-54

Impatience 108-09
Inconscience (Inconscient the) 6fn, 29, 33
  and the subconscient 6fn, 32-33
Indecision 105-106
Inner being, *see under* Being
Insanity 119
Introspection 19, 52

James, William 24-25, 122
Jung, Carl 11, 12, 13, 24, 26-29, 36, 39, 40, 49, 52, 59-60
  on archetypes and religion 85
  on ego 20, 117
  and Freud 11, 27-29
  on Samadhi 91-93
  and Sri Aurobindo 11, 12, 13, 39-40
  on the unconscious 11, 12, 26-27, 28, 39-40, 41, 42, 47
  on Yoga 85-94

Kant, Immanuel 24
Karma 140, 143

Leibnitz, Gottfried 24
Libido 11, 28-29, 79
Life-force, *see* Vital, the

Mania 117-18
mantra 129
Maslow, Abraham 16, 17
Masochism 81, 110, 111
Mastery 132-42 *passim*
Menninger, Karl 132
Mental (psychological) health (well-being) 56, 96-97, 132, 141
  meaning 74-76
  and spirituality 73, 83
Mind 31-32, 51, 123-24
  and consciousness 19
  connotation of 97-98
  control over 142

Index

disturbances of 76-79, 99-106
higher planes of 40-41
limitations of 41-42, 124
mental will 111-12, 123, 124, 125, 127-28, 140
mechanical 76
physical 77, 99, 103, 106
and the vital 97-98
vital mind 77, 80, 101, 102
Mother, the (quotations)
  becoming conscious 51
  circumstances 125-26, 127
  curing nervous diseases 66
  depression 79-80, 107
  desire 106-07, 110
  desire and love 63-64
  establishing peace 151-52
  fear 107
  feeling of inferiority 117
  feelings and perception 102-103
  hurry 80, 108-09, 150
  identification 61-62, 64, 65, 65-66, 66-67
  inner disharmony, nature of, and spot of body affected 116
  inner immobility 156
  parents' subconscient influence on the new-born 114-15
  physical mind 103, 104, 104-05
  positive peace 145
  psychic openness 96-97
  source of anxiety 100-01
  Tamas 111
  vibrations 154, 155
  widening of consciousness 65
  worry 78
Motivation
  forces of 11, 12
  unconscious 13
Myers F.W.H. 36

Nivedita, Sister 89
Nolini Kanta Gupta 74

Normality (normal state) 20, 120
Obsessive-compulsive neurosis 77, 105-06
Occultism 86-87
Ornstein, Robert 17, 52

Pain 148
Patanjali 85, 91, 92, 93
Patel, Chandra H. 149
Pavlov, I. 14
Peck, M. Scott 119fn
Physical (being) (consciousness), the 81, 98-99, 104, 123
  and nerves 112
  disturbances of 80-81, 111-12
  vital-physical 112
Plotinus 88
Polytheism 85, 86
Possession, *see under* Adverse Forces
Prakriti (Nature) 134, 135, 136, 138, 141, 142
Prana 11
Prenatal influences 114-15
Projection 102
Psychic (being), the 120, 128, 138, 139, 140, 141
  and psychological health 97
  meaning of the term 89 fn, 99
Psychoanalysis 5, 7, 14, 16, 51, 55
  and behaviourism 14
  and reductionism 14, 16
Psychological health, *see* Mental health
Psychology
  and self-knowledge 21
  nature and scope 18
  science of consciousness 18-19
  and yoga 21, 46, 52
Psychosomatic disorders 115-16
Psychosynthesis 50, 73, 136
Purusha 134, 135, 138-39, 141, 142

Rahe, R.H. 109

Rajas   80, 133, 135, 141
Rational-Emotive Therapy   49-50
Rationalization   77, 102
Reductionism   14, 16
Relaxation (relaxing)   144, 153
Repetition compulsion, *see under* Freud
Repression   25
Rolfing   82
Rosenman, R.H.   79, 108, 150

Sachchidananda   56
Samadhi   91-93
Sanskaras   34
Sattwa   133, 134, 135, 141
Self, the   40, 50, 82, 138, 139
   and consciousness   54-55
   and existence   54
Shiatsu   82
Skinner, B.F.   14
Sri Aurobindo (quotations)
   becoming fully self-aware   42-43
   being the mind's master   142
   circumstances   126
   complexity of nature   51
   concept of the vital   11
   connotation of mind   97-98
   consciousness   53, 54-55
   detachment   142
   ego   19, 118
   fullness of being   56, 56-57
   habit   112
   healing-power of knowledge   51
   the Inconscient and Matter   30
   knowledge by identity   62-63
   Matter, Life and Mind   30-31
   mind   41
   need to know the whole   29
   psychoanalysis   7, 8
   psychology   3, 4, 14-15, 15-16, 18
   Rajas   133, 141
   reductionism   8
   Sattwa   134, 141

Self   54
self-awareness   53-54
the subconscient   5, 6, 32-33, 33-35, 37, 113, 113-14
the subliminal   36, 37-38, 39
Tamas   80, 133
tendency to keep grief   110
the two beings   138
the vital mind   102
weakness of will   111
witness attitude   129
Stress   109, 144
Subconscient (subconscious), the   5, 6, 29, 32-35, 37, 113-15
   and the inconscient   32-33
   and the subliminal   10
   and the submental   33
Subliminal, the   10, 29, 36-41
   and the collective unconscious   12, 39-40
   as a general term   36
   and the subconscient   10
Superconscience (Superconscient), the   29, 40-41
Superego   26, 27, 47, 48, 58-59
Supermind   41, 55, 55-56fn
Surface being, *see under* Being
Sutich, Anthony   17

Tamas (inertia)   111, 133, 135, 141
Titchener, E.B.   3, 18
Transactional Analysis   48-49
Transpersonal Psychology   17, 42, 46
Type A behaviour   80, 108, 150

Unconscious, the   5, 24-44 *passim*, 90, 91
   collective   11, 12, 26-27, 28, 34, 40, 47
   personal   11, 26

Vibrations   153-55

Index

Vital, the (life force) (life nature)   11, 31, 123, 124
   and the mind   97-98
   disturbances of   79-80, 106-10
   free expression of   110
   masochistic tendency of   110
   physical   99
Vital envelope   146
Vital-physical, the, *see under* Physical, the
Vivekananda   89

Watson, J.B.   13
Welwood, John   21, 25
Widening (oneself) (consciousness)   65, 153
Wilber, Ken   19, 20, 52, 53
Will, *see* mental will *under* Mind
Witness attitude   129; *cf.* Detachment
Wundt, Wilhelm   3

Yoga   21, 85, 96
   Integral Yoga   73, 75, 76, 79, 82, 83
   and mental health   73-83
   and psychology, *see under* Psychology
   and psychotherapy   51, 55, 137
   Raja Yoga, *see* Patanjali